90-DAY
GLUTEN FREE
SMART DIET
1200-CALORIE

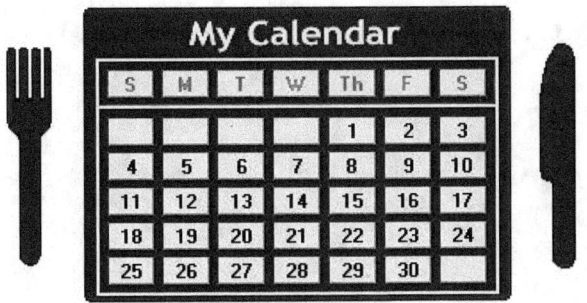

Susan Chen
Gail Johnson, M.S.

NoPaperPress™

<u>Note</u>: At publication, the off-the-shelf foods used in this book were widely available in most supermarkets. But food products come and go. So if there is a frozen entrée or soup selection in this diet that is out of stock, or that's been discontinued, or perhaps you don't like, or that you forgot to pick up while shopping, please substitute another food that has **<u>approximately</u>** the same caloric value and nutritional content. In this regard, many dieters have found the foods listed in the Appendices at the end of this book to be very helpful.

CONTENTS

Day 13 – Pasta with Marinara Sauce (123)
Day 14 - Smoothie
Day 15 – London Broil (125)
Day 16 – Baked Red Snapper
Day 17 – Cajun Chicken Salad (127)
Day 18 – Grilled Swordfish
Day 19 – Chinese Dinner Out Guidelines (129)
Day 20 – Quick Pasta Puttanesca
Day 21 - Frozen Dinner (131)
Day 22 – Shrimp & Spinach Salad
Day 23 – Beans & Greens Salad (134)
Day 24 – Four Beans Plus Salad
Day 25 – Pan-Broiled Hanger Steak (136)
Day 26 – Grilled Scallops & Polenta
Day 27 – Fettuccine in Summer Sauce (138)
Day 28 – Frozen Chicken Dinner
Day 29 – Barbequed Shrimp & Corn (141)
Day 30 – Cheeseburger Heaven
Day 31 – Baked Sea Bass (143)
Day 32 – Grilled Turkey Tenders
Day 33 – Frozen Dinner (145)
Day 34 – Pasta Rapini
Day 35 – Chicken Dinner Out (148)
Day 36 – Grilled Tilapia
Day 37 – Lo-Cal Beef Stew (151)
Day 38 – Broiled Lamb Chop
Day 39 – Chicken with Veggies (153)
Day 40 – Fish Dinner Out
Day 41 – Pasta e Fagioli (155)
Day 42 – Muffins
Day 43 – Beef Kebob (157)
Day 44 – Baked Haddock
Day 45 – Chicken Cacciatore (159)
Day 46 – Poached Cod
Day 47 – Chinese Dinner Out (161)
Day 48 – Healthy Pasta Salad
Day 49 – Frozen Dinner (163)
Day 50 – Pan-Fried Sole
Day 51 – Beans & Greens Salad (166)

Day 52 – Chicken Piccata
Day 53 – Beef Steak Strips (168)
Day 54 – Grilled Scallops & Polenta
Day 55 – Hearty Vegetable Soup (170)
Day 56 – Frozen Dinner
Day 57 – Salmon with Mango Salsa (173)
Day 58 – Grilled Pork Chop with Orange
Day 59 – Fish Dinner Out (175)
Day 60 – Chicken Stew over Rice
Day 61 – Shrimp over Spaghetti (177)
Day 62 – Beef Burgundy
Day 63 – Chicken Cutlet (179)
Day 64 – Personal-Size Meat Loaf
Day 65 – Frozen Dinner (181)
Day 66 – Pepper & Mushroom Pizza
Day 67 – Chicken Dinner Out (184)
Day 68 – Pork Medallions in Lime Sauce
Day 69 – Healthy Chicken Salad (187)
Day 70 – Baked Cod
Day 71 – Chicken Scaloppini (189)
Day 72 – Fish Dinner Out
Day 73 – Pasta Pomodoro (191)
Day 74 – Frozen Dinner
Day 75 – Szechuan Noodles & Pork (194)
Day 76 – Grilled Scallops
Day 77 – Chicken with Peppers & Rice (196)
Day 78 – Trout with Lemon & Capers
Day 79 – Chinese Dinner Out (198)
Day 80 – Vegetable Chilli
Day 81 – Frozen Dinner (200)
Day 82 – Chinese Chicken Salad
Day 83 – Hearty Lentil Stew (203)
Day 84 – Turkey Burger
Day 85 – Lo-Cal Meat Loaf (205)
Day 86 – Tuna & Bean Salad
Day 87 – Pasta Primavera (207)
Day 88 – Frozen Dinner
Day 89 – Fish Stew (210)
Day 90 – Veal with Mushrooms & Tomato

Gluten is a mixture of two proteins that are present in wheat, barley and rye. Gluten causes harmful reactions to people who have celiac disease or are gluten sensitive. But gluten is difficult to avoid, because wheat is the third largest crop in the U.S. (behind corn and soybeans). When the acreage for wheat, barley and rye are combined, more farm acres are used to grow gluten grain crops than any other, with about 4 billion bushels of gluten grains grown in 2011. Because wheat, barley and rye grains are everywhere in our food chain, eating gluten-free is more complicated than just substituting gluten-free bread for the usual gluten-containing bread that is for sale on supermarket shelves.

Another problem is gluten cross contamination which occurs when a gluten-free food comes in contact with a food that contains gluten. Cross contamination can happen at a farm where the food is grown, at a manufacturing facility where the food is processed, at a supermarket where a food may be re-packaged, and in your kitchen.

Gluten-free means that a food does not contain the gluten in wheat, barley or rye and sometimes cross-contaminated oats or soy.

Why Gluten Free?

The primary reason for a gluten-free diet is to combat celiac disease which is a chronic, systemic, autoimmune disorder that causes intestinal damage. For more on celiac disease see **Appendix A** (page 212).

Another reason to go gluten free is to combat a condition called non-celiac gluten sensitivity that can also affect nearly every system in your body with symptoms that include digestive complaints, skin problems, brain fog, joint pain and numbness in extremities. Still another reason for a gluten-free diet is to combat a wheat allergy. For more on non-celiac gluten sensitivity see Appendix A.

A new reason to go gluten free is that many adults claim that going gluten free not only helped them lose weight but they also felt a lot better. For more on this again see Appendix A.

Is This Diet For You?

The *90-Day Gluten-Free Smart Diet - 1200 Calorie* is for adults:
- **With celiac disease who want to lose weight.**
- **With gluten sensitivity or a wheat allergy who want to lose weight.**
- **Who just want to lose weight and feel better on a gluten-free diet.**
The 1200-Calorie menus assure that you will lose weight, while going gluten free is a healthy bonus that also makes many people feel better while on the diet.

Why a 90-Day Diet?

Experts agree that a diet that promotes weight loss over a relatively longer time period is healthier and the weight loss is more likely to be more permanent. And most medical practitioners advise their patients to choose a nutritious diet that promotes a weight loss of approximately 2 pounds per week – which amounts to about 26 lbs in 90 days. The *90-Day Gluten-Free Smart Diet* fits the bill!

Expected Weight Loss

On the *90-Day Gluten-Free Smart Diet – 1200 Calorie Edition*, **most women lose 23 to 34 pounds.** Smaller women, older women and less active women lose a bit less and larger women, younger women and more active women often lose much more.

On the *90-Day Gluten-Free Smart Diet – 1200 Calorie Edition*, **most men lose 35 to 45 pounds**. Smaller men, older men and less active men will lose a tad less and larger men, younger men and more active men frequently lose much more.

Exactly how much weight you will lose depends on how much you weigh, your age and your activity level. For the full story see *Weight Loss for Men - U.S. Edition* by Vincent W. Antonetti, Ph.D., or *Weight Loss for Women - U.S. Edition* by Vincent W. Antonetti, Ph.D., also published by NoPaperPress.

Smart Diet Info

The *90-Day Gluten-Free Smart Diet* contains meal plans, recipes and guidance for 90 fat-melting days! How long you stay on the diet, 10 days, 45 days, or all 90 days – depends on how much weight you want to lose. **Day 1** of the diet starts on page 18. Associated with each of the 90 days is a "**Recipe of the Day**" on page 109 and a "Diet Tip of the Day."

First a Medical Exam

Even though the *90-Day Gluten-Free Smart Diet* adheres to the United States Department of Agriculture balanced diet recommendations, this diet may not be appropriate for everyone, such as individuals with illnesses such as heart disease, diabetes, etc. Make sure you check with your
physician before starting this diet, or any diet. **Everyone should at the very least have a medical assessment, or exam, before starting a weight loss diet.** Why? You need to make sure your health will allow you to lower your caloric intake and increase your physical activity.

Depending on your age and state of health, the medical checkup may be as simple as a visit to a physician who is familiar with your medical history, or it may be a thorough physical exam.

The physician conducting the medical exam should be made aware of and should approve the specific weight loss diet you're planning. Additionally, if you are going to engage in some sort of physical activity in conjunction with this diet and especially if you have been totally inactive, or if you have or suspect you have cardiovascular disease or other health problems, or if you are obese, or if you are 40 or older, before embarking on the physical fitness portion of your weight control program you should have a stress test supervised by a physician. Finally, your physician can tell you how much and what type of exercise is right for you, how much you should weigh, and prescribe a realistic weight-loss goal.

Eat Smart – Gluten Free

First, please read **Appendix B** "Gluten-Free Foods" on page 215 which is a listing of many of the gluten-free foods that are available in supermarkets and online.

Then understand that no single food can supply all the nutrients you need in the amounts you need. Gluten free aside for the moment, the most important factors in nutrition are variety, variety, variety! **Variety is the key to a nutritious diet.** As a means of setting strategies for food selection, the U.S. Department of Health and Human Services and the Department of Agriculture issue Dietary Guidelines every five years. The latest Dietary Guidelines describe a healthy diet as one that:
- Emphasizes fruits, vegetables, whole grains, and fat-free or low-fat milk products.
- Includes fish, poultry, lean meats, beans and nuts.
- Is low in saturated fats, trans fats, cholesterol, salt (sodium) and added sugars.

The latest guidelines encourage adults to consume a variety of nutrient-dense foods and beverages within their caloric needs. The afore mentioned U.S. government agencies recommend how much should be eaten from each of the basic food groups.

Even though most adults can get all the vitamins and minerals they need by merely consuming a variety of nutritious foods (from the fruit group, the vegetable group, the grains group, the meat and beans group, the milk group, and the oils group), many physicians recommend a daily multi-vitamin/mineral supplement – just in case you don't eat the way you should.

Be aware that some micronutrients, such as the fat-soluble vitamin A, can be harmful if taken in large quantities. To be safe your multi-vitamin/mineral supplement should contain no more than 100 percent of the recommended dietary allowance (RDA) for each vitamin or mineral. Generally, you don't need the high doses in multi-vitamin/mineral supplements labeled "therapeutic" or "extra-strength." There may be medical reasons for taking larger amounts of a vitamin or mineral than the RDA provides, but check with your doctor first.

Tossed Salad

One of the dinner mainstays in the *90-Day Gluten-Free Smart Diet* is a "Tossed Salad." To prepare your "Tossed Salad" start with a bowl that has a volume of <u>at least</u> 16 ounces, or 2 cups. First add about 1 cup of either green-leaf lettuce, Romaine lettuce or a Mesclun mix. Then add at least a half cup of other veggies such as broccoli, celery, cucumber, spinach, or watercress. This vegetable combination will, on average, total about 35 Calories.

You'll be eating a "Tossed Salad" just about every day at dinnertime. Remember that variety is the key to a nutritious diet. So be sure to vary the ingredients of the salad. Top your "Tossed Salad" with <u>1½ tablespoons of a gluten-free lite salad dressing</u> that contains no more than 25 Calories per tablespoon. Some of our favorite gluten-free light salad dressings are:
- **Annie's Lite Raspberry Vinaigrette**
- **Ken's Lite Options Italian w/ Romano & Red Pepper**
- **Newman's Own Lite Red Wine Vinaigrette & Olive Oil**
- **San-J's Tamari Sesame Salad Dressing**

For more gluten-free salad dressing options see page 222. Your "Tossed Salad" with gluten-free salad dressing will cost you roughly 70 Calories but will be packed with lots of health-giving vitamins, minerals and fiber.

About Bread

First appreciate that bread, more specifically whole-grain breads, are good sources of complex carbohydrates and dietary fiber, as well as the

B vitamins (thiamin, riboflavin, niacin, and folate), vitamin E, and minerals (iron, magnesium and selenium). The gluten in wheat, barley and rye consists of two proteins that combine during baking to develop a substance that provides bread with elasticity and structure. Gluten also helps bread dough rise into a light loaf. Other grains do not have these characteristics, which is why it is difficult to find good gluten-free bread.

The 90-*Day Gluten-Free Smart Diet* requires bread at about 70 Calories per slice. These days many supermarkets stock gluten-free bread. The difficult part is finding a good tasting gluten-free bread with about 70 Calories per slice. The gluten-free breads at your local supermarket vary in taste and texture, so try different brands before deciding. As of this writing, our favorite gluten-free bread is Udi's, particularly Udi's Whole-Grain Bread at about 65 Calories per slice.

Substituting Foods

If there is a food listed in the *90-Day Gluten-Free Smart Diet* that you don't like, or perhaps that you forgot to pick up while shopping, you probably can exchange or substitute another food in its place – a technique used by dieticians. Exchanging a food listed in a diet for another food with approximately equal caloric value and nutritional content is the foundation of many successful long-term diets. Substitution possibilities are almost endless but have to be done carefully. The easiest substitutions are those within the same food group, such as exchanging one vegetable variety for another, or a glass of milk for a cup of yogurt. More sophisticated exchanges cross food groups, such as replacing 3½ ounces of turkey with a tablespoon of peanut butter on a piece of whole-wheat bread. Both foods are complete protein and both contain about 175 Calories. With some understanding and experience, you can substitute foods called for in the *90-Day Gluten-Free Smart Diet* with equal calorie foods from the same food group.

Breakfast: You may substitute any cereal for any other gluten-free cereal. For example, if you're not crazy about having Kellogg's Rice Krispies - gluten-free for breakfast on Day 4, substitute General Mills Corn Chex, etc. Remember to adjust the amount of cereal to account for the calorie difference between brands. (See page 216 for a list of gluten-free cereals.) And if you don't like the soft-boiled egg called for on Day 9, cook a fried egg instead. And if Cantaloupe is on the menu but is not in season, replace cantaloupe with a half cup of orange juice – both contain about 50 Calories.

Snacks: Again, where 6 ounces of yogurt is specified you may substitute an 8-ounce glass of skim milk, but to maintain a nutritionally balanced diet keep this snack a dairy selection. Similarly, when fruit is on the menu, you may select any type of fruit but do not stray from the fruit group. Nuts and popcorn can be interchanged at will. Specified convenient brand-name snacks, such as Skinny Cow ice cream bars and Orville Redenbacher's Smart Pop Popcorn should be widely available but other equivalent brands may be substituted if need be. Just make sure the substitute snack has the same calorie count, or very close, to the specified snack.

Two Nights – No Cooking

Everyone deserves a break from the grind of preparing dinner after coming home from work. So the *90-Day Gluten-Free Smart Diet* gives you two days off almost every week! One night a week the meal plan calls for a frozen dinner and on a second night you are encouraged to eat out. There are, however, some rules and caveats involved – these are covered in the next two sections.

Frozen Dinner Rules

In general, a frozen dinner should not be a meal in itself. Make sure you add a salad, fruit, gluten-free bread etc. The frozen dinner you choose should come with at least one cup of cooked vegetables. If your frozen dinner doesn't measure up, add your own frozen, fresh or canned vegetables. And look for dinners with no more than 800 mg of sodium. Some reasonably good gluten-free frozen dinner choices are:
- Amy's Thai Stir-Fry (310 Calories, 420 mg sodium)
- Amy's Asian Noodle Stir Fry (300 Calories, 630 mg sodium)
- Artisan Bistro Wild Alaskan Salmon (200 Calories, 135 mg sodium)
- Artisan Bistro Savory Turkey (330 Calories, 450 mg sodium)
- Smart Ones Lemon Herb Chicken Piccata (250 Calories, 540 mg sodium)
- Smart Ones Santa Fe Style Rice & Beans (290 Calories, 660 mg sodium)
For more frozen dinner choices see **Appendix B** on page 215. On days when frozen dinner is specified, you will be given a calorie goal for the frozen dinner. For example, Day 5 calls for frozen dinner with a maximum allowable 340 Calories. If you choose a frozen dinner that contains less than 340 Calories, you may spend the unused calories any way you wish.

Moreover, on those nights when you just don't have the energy or time to cook, you can always substitute a frozen dinner for the "Recipe of the Day" or the entree listed in the meal plan. Again the substitute food should be close in calorie value to the food it replaces.

Eating Out Challenges

You may eat out once a week. When you're on a gluten-free reducing diet, however, eating in a restaurant can be a double challenge. First, most
restaurant portions are huge, easily totaling more than 1,000 Calories, and then many restaurants do not offer gluten-free menu selections. On the *90-Day Gluten-Free Smart Diet*, a dinner type (i.e., fish, chicken, etc) and a calorie target are specified. For example Day 7 of the 1,200 Calorie diet calls for a chicken dinner and allows you 530 Calories. Follow these tips to make sure your dinning experience is both low calorie, gluten-free and pleasant.

Make sure you choose a restaurant where gluten-free food is available and where you have a fighting chance to achieve your calorie goal. Before you go read the menu online and reduce your food choices so you can have more focused questions for the staff. You are more likely to get a safe meal if you call the restaurant before you go to let them know of your gluten-free needs. And call during a slow time so you can have the host's complete attention.

In the restaurant, to ensure you are served a gluten-free meal, it is important to communicate your need to eat 100 percent gluten-free assertively but amiably. Try to speak directly to the chef or manager. Otherwise, ask your server what is in the food and how it's prepared. Menu descriptions don't always list every ingredient. Try to get a list of ingredients for sauces and dressings. Inquire how gluten-free grains such as rice and risottos are cooked. Sometimes they are cooked in broth which may contain gluten. Confirm that separate, clean utensils and equipment will be used to prepare your meal.

Order something simple, such as broiled fish with steamed vegetables and brown rice. Tell the waiter you want no sauce, no gravy, nothing added. Then, knowing your calorie objective, and that most fish and chicken are about 50 Calories per ounce, most steamed vegetable servings average approximately 50 Calories per cup, and rice is about 100 Calories per ½ cup, decide how much to eat – and take the

13

remainder home. And consider bringing your own gluten-free salad dressing to the restaurant. If fresh fruit is not an option, pass on dessert and have the evening snack specified in the *90-Day Gluten-Free Smart Diet* meal plan for that day.

   Eating Chinese can be especially difficult. Try bringing a restaurant card to the Chinese restaurant. The cards are available online and are designed to help explain a gluten-free diet to a waiter who might not speak English. Rice noodles prepared with vegetables or chicken are generally a safe choice. If you have celiac disease or non-celiac gluten sensitivity, avoid brown sauce which may have a cross-contaminated soy sauce base. Instead, ask for the dish to be prepared with a white sauce using corn starch. And although it is customary to share dishes at a Chinese restaurant, do not permit your dinner companions to contaminate your food. Make sure your friends do not use their gluten-contaminated spoons to serve food from your gluten-free dish.

   Social Gatherings can be tricky. At a dinner party, intermingling utensils and serving dishes create a perfect environment for gluten cross contamination, that is for gluten to get in your food. But this does not necessarily mean you should to skip the party. Try to let your host know ahead of time about your gluten-free needs. Do this before your host starts planning the menu. Even better, offer to bring a few dishes to share. This ensures that there will be at least a couple of items you can eat safely and takes a burden off of your host. Finally, ask the host if you can serve yourself first, before serving plates become gluten contaminated.

Smart Diet Notes

1) Coffee or tea may be regular or decaf. If desired, skim milk and a sugar substitute may be added to coffee or tea.

2) Fried eggs and scrambled eggs should be cooked in a pan coated with a non-stick cooking spray. DO NOT USE butter or oil.

3) On bread, corn-on-the-cob, or a baked potato, if desired, you may use a zero-calorie butter substitute spray. (I Can't Believe It's Not Butter spray is gluten free.) DO NOT USE butter or sour cream.

4) Cereals should be selected from the following gluten-free varieties: General Mills Rice Chex, General Mills Corn Chex, General Mills Vanilla Chex, General Mills Cinnamon Chex, General Mills Chocolate Chex, General Mills Apple Cinnamon Chex, General Mills Honey Nut Chex, Glutino Honey Nut, Glutino Apple Cinnamon, Kellogg's Rice

Krispies - gluten-free, Bob's Red Mill Oat Meal and Gifts of Nature (Montana) Oat Meal. When blueberries are in season, you may **substitute blueberries for raisins** added to your cereal. (Substitution ratio = 2 blueberries per raisin.)

5) Bread: Udi's Whole Grain Bread is a good choice and has 65 Calories per slice. These days many supermarkets stock gluten-free bread although you often can find a better selection online. If desired, bread may be sprayed with a zero-calorie butter substitute. DO NOT USE butter.

6) Use only lean cuts of meat trimmed of all visible fat. Poultry should be limited to chicken or turkey breasts (white meat and skinless only).

7) When canned fish is specified, use only fish packed in water.

8) An unlimited amount of green salad may be eaten, but the GF salad dressing should be as specified in page 10. (Note, in the meal plans Evoo means extra virgin olive oil.)

9) Use freely as desired: clear unsweetened coffee, clear unsweetened tea, water, seltzer water, any diet soda, clear soups without fat, bouillon, and seasonings such as mustard, cinnamon, dill, herbs, red and black pepper, curry and vinegar.

10) On days when a leftover is specified for lunch. Eat about half as much as you ate for dinner a night or two before.

11) Any specified snack may be moved to any other part of the day, and/or combined with lunch or dinner.

12) Although it's recommended that you follow the diet days as specified, it's fine to occasionally skip a day and/or pick and choose the days you prefer. (Nutritionally, each day stands on its own.)

13) After you complete the 90th day on the diet, if you still want to lose more weight you may repeat the diet by starting over at Day 1.

Keeping It Off

Within five years, more than 90 percent of all dieters regain every pound they have lost. Why? In most cases it's because after losing weight most people eventually revert to their pre-diet eating and exercising habits, and this inevitably leads to their regaining the weight they lost – and often more. Obviously after a diet you weigh less. The fact is the less you weigh, the less you need to eat to sustain your lower weight.

A study, published in the *Annals of Internal Medicine*, that followed 4,000 people for three decades suggests that in the long term,

90 percent of men and 70 percent of women will become overweight. Interestingly, half of the men and women in the study, who had made it well into adulthood without a weight problem, ultimately also became overweight and a third actually became obese. The point being that you can never become complacent. You must continually watch your weight because we are all at risk of becoming overweight.

The key to long-term weight control success is knowledge and understanding, combined of course with desire and self-discipline. Once you reach your weight goal, we suggest you read *Weight Maintenance - U.S. Edition* by Vincent Antonetti, Ph.D. (also published by NoPaperPress) – absolutely the best weight maintenance book on the market.

1200 Calorie Daily Menus

Day 1 - 1200 Calorie Meal Plan

BREAKFAST	Calories	Totals
Grapefruit (½)	**75**	
Scrambled egg	**80**	
Gluten-free bread (See page 216**) toasted (1 slice)**	**70**	
Coffee (See Notes page 14**)**	**10**	**235 Cal**
SNACK		
Coffee or tea	**10**	**10 Cal**
LUNCH		
Ham (See page 220**) (2 oz) w mustard 2 slices GF bread**	**290**	
Pickle spear	**0**	
Small bunch of grapes	**65**	
Hot or iced tea	**10**	**365 Cal**
SNACK		
Fresh fruit in season (apple, peach, etc)	**70**	
Coffee or tea	**10**	**80 Cal**
DINNER		
Chicken w Peppers & Onions **(**Day 1 Recipe page 109**)**	**250**	
Sautéed red peppers with onions (Day 1 recipe)	**70**	
Green beans - steamed	**25**	
Mashed cauliflower	**30**	
Large tossed salad 1½ Tbsp lite GF dressing (page 222)	**70**	
Water	**0**	**445 Cal**
SNACK		
GF Cookie (page 218)	**60**	
Coffee or tea	**10**	**70 Cal**
		1205 Cal

Day 2 1200 Calorie Meal Plan

BREAKFAST	Calories	Totals
Orange juice (½ cup)	50	
Rice Chex* (1 cup) + ½ cup skim milk + ½ banana	195	
Coffee	10	255 Cal
* See page 216 for more GF cereals.		
SNACK		
Fresh fruit in season (apple, pear, etc)	70	
Coffee or tea	10	80 Cal
LUNCH		
GF Soup (Appendix C - page 225)	110	
Turkey breast (page 220) (1 oz on 1 slice GF bread)	120	
Pickle spear	0	
Lettuce & tomato slices	20	
Water	0	250 Cal
SNACK		
Coffee or tea	10	10 Cal
DINNER		
Baked Herb-Crusted Cod (Day 2 Recipe - page 110)	230	
Spinach (½ cup) steamed with garlic & drizzled	100	
Asparagus (8 spears cooked & drained)	25	
Baked potato (medium - No Butter!)	100	
Gluten-free (1 slice) (See page 216)	70	
Water with lemon wedge	10	535 Cal
SNACK		
GF Cookie	60	
Coffee or tea	10	70 Cal
		1200 Cal

Day 3 1200 Calorie Meal Plan

BREAKFAST	Calories	Totals
Fresh or frozen strawberries (½ cup)	25	
French toast (Day 3 Recipe - page 111)	310	
GF Lite Syrup - page 224 (1 Tbsp)	30	
Coffee	10	375 Cal
SNACK		
Coffee or tea	10	10 Cal
LUNCH		
Salad (3 oz canned tuna (page 221) 1 tsp Evoo, onions, celery)	175	
Lettuce & tomato wedges	20	
GF bread - page 216 (1 slice)	70	
Fresh fruit in season (apple, plum, etc)	70	
Coffee or tea	10	345 Cal
SNACK		
Coffee or tea	10	10 Cal
DINNER		
Broiled veal chop (4 oz lean)	200	
Corn on the cob (1 medium ear) (No Butter!)	100	
Broccoli (½ cup steamed & drizzled with 1 tsp	70	
Large tossed salad w 1½ Tbsp lite GF dressing - page 222	70	
Water with lemon wedge	10	450 Cal
SNACK		
Coffee or tea	10	10 Cal
		1200 Cal

Day 4 1200 Calorie Meal Plan

BREAKFAST	Calorie	Totals
Grapefruit (½)	75	
Rice Krispies* (1 cup) + ½ cup skim milk + about 15 raisins	200	
Coffee	10	285 Cal
* Gluten-free variety		
SNACK		
Coffee or tea	10	10 Cal
LUNCH		
GF Cottage cheese (1 cup no fat) - See page 222	140	
Tossed salad w 1½ Tbsp lite GF dressing - page 222	70	
GF bread (1 slice)	70	
Hot or iced tea	10	290 Cal
Note: Cabot No-Fat Cottage Cheese is gluten free		
SNACK		
Fresh fruit in season (peach, plum, etc)	70	
Coffee or tea	10	80 Cal
DINNER		
Meat Loaf (Day 4 Recipe - page 112)	290	
One-half acorn squash (baked with ½ tsp maple	90	
Spinach (½ cup steamed & drizzled with 1 tsp Evoo)	70	
Romaine lettuce, tomato slices & 1 Tbsp lite GF dressing	45	
Water	0	495 Cal
Note: Pure maple syrup is naturally gluten free		
SNACK		
GF Ginger-Snap Cookie - page 218	40	
Coffee or tea	10	50 Cal
See page 15 re substituting blueberries for raisins.		1210 Cal

Day 5 1200 Calorie Meal Plan

BREAKFAST	Calories	Totals
Orange juice (½ cup)	50	
Fried egg	80	
Toasted GF raisin bread (1 slice) - page 216	70	
Coffee	10	210 Cal
SNACK		
Coffee or tea	10	10 Cal
LUNCH		
GF Soup (Appendix C - page 225)	150	
GF bread (1 slice)	70	
Lettuce and sliced tomato with 1 Tbsp lite GF	45	
Canned pineapple (½ cup, no-sugar-added juice)	40	
Water	0	305 Cal
SNACK		
GF Yogurt (6 oz, non-fat, any flavor)*	90	
Coffee or tea	10	100 Cal
DINNER		
Frozen dinner (Day 5 Recipe - page 113)	340	
Large tossed salad with 1½ Tbsp lite GF dressing	70	
GF bread (1 slice)	70	
Fresh fruit in season (apple, peach, etc)	70	
Hot or iced tea	10	560 Cal
SNACK		
Coffee or tea	10	10 Cal
* Such as Yoplait Light which is non-fat & gluten free.		1200 Cal

Day 6 1200 Calorie Meal Plan

BREAKFAST	Calories	Totals
Orange juice (½ cup)	50	
GF Cinnamon Chex (¾ cup) + ½ cup skim milk + ½ banana	215	
Coffee	10	275 Cal
SNACK		
Fresh fruit in season (apple, plum, etc)	70	
Coffee or tea	10	80 Cal
LUNCH		
Leftover meat loaf (½ of Day 4 serving size)	155	
GF bread (1 slice)	70	
Lettuce	10	
Fresh or frozen berries (½ cup)	50	
Hot or iced tea	10	295 Cal
SNACK		
Handful unsalted mixed nuts (Nuts are naturally GF.)	100	
Coffee or tea	10	110 Cal
DINNER		
Margherita Pizza (Day 6 Recipe - page 115)	230	
Large tossed salad with 1½ Tbsp lite GF dressing	70	
Water with lemon wedge	10	310 Cal
SNACK		
Skinny Cow Chocolate Truffle Bar**	100	
Coffee or tea	10	110 Cal
** All Skinny Cow ice cream products are GF.		1180 Cal

Day 7 1200 Calorie Meal Plan

BREAKFAST	Calories	Totals
Cantaloupe (½ medium)	50	
GF Oatmeal* (½ cup dry) + ½ cup skim milk + about 15 raisins	230	
Coffee	10	290 Cal
* See page 216.		
SNACK		
Coffee or tea	10	10 Cal
LUNCH		
GF Soup (Appendix C - page 225)	80	
Grilled cheese sandwich (2 slices GF light cheese)*	270	
Lettuce and sliced tomato	20	
Pickle spear	0	
Water	0	370 Cal
* Most cheeses are GF. (Sandwich has 2 slices GF bread.)		
SNACK		
Coffee or tea	10	10 Cal
DINNER		
Eat Out - Chicken dinner (Day 7 Recipe - page 116)		
Max allowable calories	530	530 Cal
SNACK		
Coffee or tea	10	10 Cal
		1220 Cal

Day 8 1200 Calorie Meal Plan

BREAKFAST	Calories	Totals
Cantaloupe (½ medium)	50	
GF Rice Chex (1 cup) + ½ cup skim milk + ½ banana	195	
Coffee	10	255 Cal
SNACK		
Fresh fruit in season (peach, plum, etc)	70	
Coffee or tea	10	80 Cal
LUNCH		
GF Soup (Appendix C - page 225)	140	
Turkey breast* (1 oz) on 1 slice GF bread (½ sandwich)	120	
Lettuce & tomato slices	20	
Hot or iced tea	10	290 Cal
* See page 220		
SNACK		
Coffee or tea	10	10 Cal
DINNER		
Baked salmon with salsa (Day 8 Recipe - page 118)	215	
Baked summer squash and zucchini	40	
Medium tomato - sliced	20	
Brown rice (½ cup – after cooking)	100	
Large tossed salad with 1½ Tbsp lite GF dressing	70	
Water	0	445 Cal
SNACK		
Popcorn Mini Bag*	100	
Coffee or tea	10	110 Cal
* Such as Orville Redenbacher's Smart Pop		1200 Cal

Day 9 1200 Calorie Meal Plan

BREAKFAST	Calories	Totals
Orange juice (½ cup)	50	
Soft-boiled egg	80	
GF bread toasted (1 slice)	70	
Coffee	10	210 Cal
SNACK		
GF Yogurt (6 oz)*	90	
Coffee or tea	10	100 Cal
LUNCH		
Salad (3 oz canned tuna (page 221) 1 tsp Evoo, onions, celery)	175	
Lettuce & tomato wedges + GF bread (1 slice)	90	
Coffee or tea	10	275 Cal
SNACK		
Handful unsalted mixed nuts	100	
Coffee or tea	10	110 Cal
DINNER		
Veggie burger – (1 patty) (Day 9 Recipe - page 119)	110	
Light GF cheese slice (1 oz)	70	
GF Burger Bun - page 216	180	
Beets (3 small, boiled, skinned & sliced)	45	
Fresh fruit in season (apple, peach, etc)	70	
Water	0	475 Cal
SNACK		
Coffee or tea	10	10 Cal
* Such as Yoplait Light which is non-fat & gluten free.		1180 Cal

Day 10 1200 Calorie Meal Plan

BREAKFAST	Calories	Totals
Orange juice (½ cup)	50	
Wild blueberry pancakes (Day 10 Recipe - page 120)	210	
GF Lite Syrup (1½ Tbsp) - page 224	45	
Coffee	10	315 Cal
SNACK		
Coffee or tea	10	10 Cal
LUNCH		
GF Peanut butter (2 Tbsp) on 2 slices of GF bread - page 222	330	
Skim milk (4 oz)	45	
Fresh fruit in season (apple, plum, etc)	70	
Water	0	445 Cal
SNACK		
Coffee or tea	10	10 Cal
DINNER		
Broiled pork chop (about 4 oz meat - trimmed of fat)	280	
Green peas (½ cup)	55	
Tomato & cucumber salad w 1½ Tbsp GF dressing	70	
Water with lemon wedge	10	415 Cal
SNACK		
Coffee or tea	10	10 Cal
		1205 Cal

Day 11 1200 Calorie Meal Plan

BREAKFAST	Calories	Totals
Fresh sliced orange	75	
Rice Krispies* (1 cup) + ½ cup skim milk + about 15 raisins	200	
Coffee	10	285 Cal
* Gluten free variety		
SNACK		
Coffee or tea	10	10 Cal
LUNCH		
GF Cottage cheese* (1 cup no fat)	140	
Large tossed salad with 1½ Tbsp lite GF dressing	70	
GF bread (1 slice)	70	
Hot or iced tea	10	290 Cal
* Cabot No-Fat Cottage Cheese is gluten free		
SNACK		
Handful unsalted mixed nuts	100	
Coffee or tea	10	110 Cal
DINNER		
GF chicken sausage* (2 links about 2½ oz per link)	180	
Artichoke-bean salad (Day 11 Recipe - page 121)	190	
Green beans (¼ lb – steamed)	25	
GF bread (1 slice)	70	
Water	0	465 Cal
SNACK		
GF Ginger-Snap Cookie - page 218	40	
Coffee or tea	10	50 Cal
* See page 221.		1210 Cal

Day 12 1200 Calorie Meal Plan

BREAKFAST	Calories	Totals
Orange juice (½ cup)	50	
Scrambled egg	80	
GF bread toasted (1 slice)	70	
Coffee	10	210 Cal
SNACK		
GF Yogurt (6 oz)	90	
Coffee or tea	10	100 Cal
LUNCH		
GF Soup (Appendix C - page 225)	150	
Tomato slices with ¼ cup chopped fresh basil + 1 tsp Evoo	60	
GF bread (1 slice)	70	
Hot or iced tea	10	290 Cal
SNACK		
Coffee or tea	10	10 Cal
DINNER		
Eat Out – Fish dinner (Day 12 Recipe - page 122)		
Max allowable calories	595	595 Cal
SNACK		
Coffee or tea	10	10 Cal
		1215 Cal

Day 13 1200 Calorie Meal Plan

BREAKFAST	Calories	Totals
Orange juice (½ cup)	50	
Cinnamon Chex (1 cup) + ½ cup skim milk + ½ banana	255	
Coffee	10	315 Cal
SNACK		
Handful unsalted mixed nuts	100	
Coffee or tea	10	110 Cal
LUNCH		
GF Turkey Hot Dog w mustard & relish - page 221	100	
GF Hot-dog bun - page 216	150	
Diet soda (or water)	0	250 Cal
SNACK		
Coffee or tea	10	10 Cal
DINNER		
Pasta with Marinara sauce (Day 13 Recipe - page 123)	225	
Large tossed salad with 1½ Tbsp lite GF dressing	70	
Fresh fruit in season (peach, plum, etc)	70	
GF bread (1 slice)	70	
Water with lemon wedge	10	445 Cal
SNACK		
GF Cookie - page 218	60	
Coffee or tea	10	70 Cal
		1200 Cal

Day 14 1200 Calorie Meal Plan

BREAKFAST	Calories	Totals
Cantaloupe (½ medium)	50	
Low-Cal Smoothie (Day 14 Recipe - page 124)	220	
Coffee	10	280 Cal
SNACK		
Fresh fruit in season (apple, peach, etc)	70	
Coffee or tea	10	80 Cal
LUNCH		
Grilled cheese sandwich (2 slices GF light cheese)*	270	
Pickle spear	0	
Hot or iced tea	10	290 Cal
* Sandwich has 2 slices GF bread		
SNACK		
Popcorn Mini Bag	100	
Coffee or tea	10	110 Cal
DINNER		
Frozen dinner (Day 5 Recipe - page 113)	300	
Large tossed salad with 1½ Tbsp lite GF dressing	70	
Water with lemon wedge	10	380 Cal
SNACK		
GF Ginger-Snap Cookie	40	
Coffee or tea	10	50 Cal
		1190 Cal

Day 15 1200 Calorie Meal Plan

BREAKFAST	Calories	Totals
Fresh or frozen strawberries (1 cup)	50	
French toast (Day 3 Recipe - page 111)	310	
GF Lite Syrup - page 224 (1 Tbsp)	30	
Coffee	10	400 Cal
SNACK		
Coffee or tea	10	10 Cal
LUNCH		
Salad (3 oz canned tuna, 1 tsp Evoo, onions, celery)	175	
GF bread (1 slice)	70	
Water	0	245 Cal
SNACK		
Fresh fruit in season (apple, plum, etc)	70	
Coffee or tea	10	80 Cal
DINNER		
London broil (Day 15 Recipe - page 125)	320	
Brown rice* (½ cup – after cooking)	100	
Steamed broccoli (1 cup – after cooking)	50	
Water	0	470 Cal
SNACK		
Coffee or tea	10	10 Cal
* Rice is naturally gluten free.		1215 Cal

Day 16 1200 Calorie Meal Plan

BREAKFAST	Calories	Totals
Orange juice (½ cup)	50	
GF Oatmeal (½ cup dry) + ½ cup skim milk + about 15 raisins	230	
Coffee	10	290 Cal
SNACK		
Fresh fruit in season (apple, plum, etc)	70	
Coffee or tea	10	80 Cal
LUNCH		
GF Soup (Appendix C - page 225)	110	
GF bread (1 slice)	70	
Lettuce & sliced tomato with 1 Tbsp lite GF	45	
Hot or iced tea	10	235 Cal
SNACK		
Coffee or tea	10	10 Cal
DINNER		
Baked red snapper (Day 16 Recipe - page 126)	215	
Wild rice mix (Day 16 Recipe)	160	
Green beans & tomato	75	
Water with lemon wedge	10	460 Cal
SNACK		
Popcorn Mini Bag	100	
Coffee or tea	10	110 Cal
		1185 Cal

Day 17 1200 Calorie Meal Plan

BREAKFAST	Calories	Totals
Cantaloupe (½ medium)	50	
Fried egg	80	
GF raisin bread - toasted (1 slice)	75	
Coffee	10	215 Cal
SNACK		
GF Yogurt (6 oz)	90	
Coffee or tea	10	100 Cal
LUNCH		
GF Soup (Appendix C - page 225)	180	
Lettuce & tomato sandwich* (Tbsp light mayo*)	170	
Cucumber slices and carrots & celery sticks	15	
Hot or iced tea	10	375 Cal
* Sandwich made with GF bread		
SNACK		
Handful unsalted mixed nuts	100	
Coffee or tea	10	110 Cal
DINNER		
Cajun chicken salad (Day 17 Recipe - page 127)	330	
GF bread (1 slice)	70	
Water	0	400 Cal
SNACK		
Coffee or tea	10	10 Cal
* Hellmann's and Best Foods regular and lite mayo are GF.		1210 Cal

Day 18 1200 Calorie Meal Plan

BREAKFAST	Calories	Totals
Grapefruit (½)	75	
Corn Chex (1 cup) + ½ cup skim milk + ½ banana	215	
Coffee	10	300 Cal
SNACK		
Coffee or tea	10	10 Cal
LUNCH		
GF Cottage cheese* (1 cup no fat)	140	
Large tossed salad with 1½ Tbsp lite GF dressing	70	
GF bread (1 slice)	70	
Hot or iced tea	10	290 Cal
* Cabot No-Fat Cottage Cheese is GF		
SNACK		
Handful unsalted mixed nuts	100	
Coffee or tea	10	110 Cal
DINNER		
Grilled swordfish (Day 18 Recipe - page 127)	250	
Grilled potatoes (Day 18 Recipe)	100	
Grilled cherry tomatoes (Day 18 Recipe)	50	
Spinach (½ cup) steamed with garlic & drizzled	50	
Water with lemon wedge	10	460 Cal
SNACK		
Coffee or tea	10	10 Cal
		1180 Cal

Day 19 1200 Calorie Meal Plan

BREAKFAST	Calories	Totals
Grapefruit (½)	75	
Scrambled egg	80	
GF bread toasted (1 slice)	70	
Coffee	10	235 Cal
SNACK		
GF Yogurt (6 oz)	90	
Coffee or tea	10	100 Cal
LUNCH		
GF Soup (Appendix C - page 225)	100	
GF turkey breast* (1 oz) on 1 slice GF bread	120	
Water	0	220 Cal
* See page 220.		
SNACK		
Coffee or tea	10	10 Cal
DINNER		
Eat Out – Chinese food** (Day 19 Recipe - page 129)		
Max allowable calories	640	640 Cal
** Order about 900 Cal. Take home ⅓ (about 300 Cal) for lunch.		
SNACK		
Coffee or tea	10	10 Cal
		1215 Cal

Day 20 1200 Calorie Meal Plan

BREAKFAST	Calories	Totals
Orange juice (½ cup)	50	
Cream of Rice (1 packet) + ½ cup skim milk + about 15 raisins	230	
Coffee	10	290 Cal
SNACK		
Handful unsalted mixed nuts	100	
Coffee or tea	10	110 Cal
LUNCH		
Left over Chinese food from Day 19	260	
Hot or iced tea	10	270 Cal
SNACK		
Coffee or tea	10	10 Cal
DINNER		
Spaghetti alla Puttanesca (Day 20 Recipe -page 130)	345	
Large tossed salad with 1½ Tbsp lite GF dressing	70	
GF bread (1 slice)	70	
Water	0	485 Cal
SNACK		
GF Ginger-Snap Cookie	40	
Coffee or tea	10	50 Cal
		1215 Cal

Day 21 1200 Calorie Meal Plan

BREAKFAST	Calories	Totals
Cantaloupe (½ medium)	50	
Chocolate Chex (¾ cup) + ½ cup skim milk + ½ banana	225	
Coffee	10	285 Cal
SNACK		
Coffee or tea	10	10 Cal
LUNCH		
GF Turkey breast (2 oz) on 2 slices GF bread	240	
Lettuce, tomato and Tbsp GF light mayo	35	
Pickle spear	0	
Fresh fruit in season (peach, plum, etc)	70	
Water	0	345 Cal
SNACK		
Popcorn Mini Bag	100	
Coffee or tea	10	110 Cal
DINNER		
Frozen dinner (Day 21 Recipe - page 131)	300	
Large tossed salad with 1½ Tbsp lite GF dressing	70	
Water with lemon wedge	10	380 Cal
SNACK		
GF Cookie	60	
Coffee or tea	10	70 Cal
		1200 Cal

Day 22 1200 Calorie Meal Plan

BREAKFAST	Calories	Totals
Fresh or frozen strawberries (1 cup)	25	
French toast (Day 3 Recipe - page 111)	310	
GF Lite Syrup	30	
Coffee	10	375 Cal
SNACK		
Coffee or tea	10	10 Cal
LUNCH		
GF Soup (Appendix C - page 225)	110	
BLT sandwich - lettuce & tomato*	270	
Pickle spear	0	
Hot or iced tea	10	390 Cal
* 2 slices GF turkey bacon & 1 Tbsp GF light mayo		
SNACK		
Coffee or tea	10	10 Cal
DINNER		
Shrimp & spinach salad (Day 22 Recipe - page 133)	310	
GF bread (1 slice)	70	
Water with lemon wedge	10	390 Cal
SNACK		
Coffee or tea	10	10 Cal
		1185 Cal

Day 23 1200 Calorie Meal Plan

BREAKFAST	Calories	Totals
Cantaloupe (½ medium)	**50**	
Glutino Honey Nut* (¾ cup) + ½ cup skim milk + ½ banana	**215**	
Coffee	**10**	**275 Cal**
* GF Cereal or a substitute if unavailable.		
SNACK		
Handful unsalted mixed nuts	**100**	
Coffee or tea	**10**	**110 Cal**
LUNCH		
GF Ham (2 oz) with mustard on 2 slices GF bread	**290**	
Pickle spear	**0**	
Hot or iced tea	**10**	**300 Cal**
SNACK		
Fresh fruit in season (apple, plum, etc)	**70**	
Coffee or tea	**10**	**80 Cal**
DINNER		
Beans & Greens Salad (Day 23 Recipe - page 134)	**260**	
GF bread (1 slice)	**70**	
Baked potato (medium) - No butter!	**100**	
Water	**0**	**430 Cal**
SNACK		
Coffee or tea	**10**	**10 Cal**
		1205 Cal

Day 24 1200 Calorie Meal Plan

BREAKFAST	Calories	Totals
Fresh orange sliced	75	
Soft-boiled egg	80	
GF bread -toasted (1 slice)	70	
Coffee	10	235 Cal
SNACK		
GF Yogurt (6 oz)*	90	
Coffee or tea	10	100 Cal
LUNCH		
Salad – 3 oz canned salmon*, 1 tsp Evoo, onions & celery	200	
Lettuce & tomato wedges	20	
GF bread (1 slice)	70	
Coffee or tea	10	300 Cal
* Canned salmon produced by Bubble Bee is gluten free.		
SNACK		
Fresh fruit in season (peach, plum, etc)	70	
Coffee or tea	10	80 Cal
DINNER		
Chicken breast (5 oz - broiled)	250	
Four bean plus salad (½ cup) (Day 24 Recipe- page135)	135	
Large tossed salad with 1½ Tbsp lite GF dressing	70	
Water with lemon wedge	10	465 Cal
SNACK		
Coffee or tea	10	10 Cal
* Such as Yoplait Light which is non-fat & gluten free.		1190 Cal

Day 25 1200 Calorie Meal Plan

BREAKFAST	Calories	Totals
Orange juice (½ cup)	50	
Corn Chex (1 cup) + ½ cup skim milk + about 15 raisins	200	
Coffee	10	260 Cal
SNACK		
Coffee or tea	10	10 Cal
LUNCH		
GF Cottage Cheese* (1 cup no fat)	140	
Large tossed salad with 1½ Tbsp lite GF dressing	70	
GF bread (1 slice)	70	
Hot or iced tea	10	290 Cal
* Cabot No-Fat Cottage Cheese is gluten free.		
SNACK		
Coffee or tea	10	10 Cal
DINNER		
Hanger steak (Day 25 Recipe - page 136)	320	
Roasted potatoes (Day 25 Recipe)	120	
Cherry tomatoes (Day 25 Recipe)	20	
Steamed spinach (½ cup)	25	
GF bread (1 slice)	70	
Hot or iced tea	10	565 Cal
SNACK		
GF Cookie	60	
Coffee or tea	10	70 Cal
		1205 Cal

Day 26 1200 Calorie Meal Plan

BREAKFAST	Calories	Totals
Cantaloupe (½ medium)	50	
Fried eggs (2 eggs)	160	
GF bread - toasted (1 slice)	70	
Coffee	10	290 Cal
SNACK		
GF Yogurt (6 oz)	90	
Coffee or tea	10	100 Cal
LUNCH		
GF Soup (Appendix C - page 225)	160	
GF bread (1 slice)	70	
Lettuce & tomato slices	20	
Hot or iced tea	10	260 Cal
SNACK		
Fresh fruit in season (apple, peach, etc)	70	
Coffee or tea	10	80 Cal
DINNER		
Grilled scallops (Day 26 Recipe - page 137)	210	
Grilled polenta (Day 26 Recipe)	125	
Mushroom-steamed green beans-red onion	45	
Grilled asparagus	10	
Large tossed salad with 1½ Tbsp lite GF dressing	70	
Water	0	460 Cal
SNACK		
Coffee or tea	10	10 Cal
		1200 Cal

Day 27 1200 Calorie Meal Plan

BREAKFAST	Calories	Totals
Orange juice (½ cup)	50	
Cream of Rice (1 packet) + ½ cup skim milk + about 15 raisins	230	
Coffee	10	290 Cal
SNACK		
Coffee or tea	10	10 Cal
LUNCH		
Two servings (1 cup) left over bean salad from Day 24	270	
GF bread (1 slice)	70	
Lettuce & tomato slices	20	
Hot or iced tea	10	370 Cal
SNACK		
Fresh fruit in season (apple, plum, etc)	70	
Coffee or tea	10	80 Cal
DINNER		
Fettuccine (Day 27 Recipe - page 138)	290	
Large tossed salad with 1½ Tbsp lite GF dressing	70	
GF bread (1 slice)	80	
Water	0	440 Cal
SNACK		
Coffee or tea	10	10 Cal
		1200 Cal

Day 28 1200 Calorie Meal Plan

BREAKFAST	Calories	Totals
Cantaloupe (½ medium)	50	
Smoothie (Day 14 Recipe - page 124)	220	
Coffee	10	280 Cal
SNACK		
Fresh fruit in season (peach, plum, etc)	70	
Coffee or tea	10	80 Cal
LUNCH		
Roast beef (2 oz) sandwich on GF bread	295	
Lettuce	0	
Hot or iced tea	10	305 Cal
SNACK		
Coffee or tea	10	10 Cal
DINNER		
Frozen dinner (Day 28 Recipe - page 139)	300	
Large tossed salad with 1½ Tbsp lite GF dressing	70	
GF bread (1 slice)	70	
Fresh fruit in season (apple, plum, etc)	70	
Water with lemon wedge	10	520 Cal
SNACK		
Coffee or tea	10	10 Cal
		1205 Cal

Day 29 1200 Calorie Meal Plan

BREAKFAST	Calories	Totals
Orange juice (½ cup)	50	
Wild blueberry pancakes (Day 10 Recipe - page 120)	190	
GF Lite Syrup (1½ Tbsp)	45	
Coffee	10	295 Cal
SNACK		
GF Yogurt (6 oz)	90	
Coffee or tea	10	100 Cal
LUNCH		
Salad (3 oz canned tuna, 1 tsp Evoo, onions, celery)	175	
Lettuce & tomato wedges	20	
GF bread (1 slice)	70	
Fresh fruit in season (apple, pear, etc)	70	
Coffee or tea	10	345 Cal
SNACK		
Coffee or tea	10	10 Cal
DINNER		
Barbequed shrimp (Day 29 Recipe - page 141)	160	
Corn on the cob (medium)	90	
Steamed broccoli (1 cup – after cooking)	50	
Water	0	300 Cal
SNACK		
Glutino Chocolate-Covered Pretzels*	140	
Coffee or tea	10	150 Cal
* 9 pretzels		1200 Cal

Day 30 1200 Calorie Meal Plan

BREAKFAST	Calories	Totals
Fresh orange sliced	75	
Chocolate Chex (¾ cup) + ½ cup skim milk + ½ banana	225	
Coffee	10	310 Cal
SNACK		
Fresh fruit in season (apple, plum, etc)	70	
Coffee or tea	10	80 Cal
LUNCH		
GF Soup (Appendix C - page 225)	150	
GF bread (1 slice)	70	
Raw zucchini slices, celery & carrot sticks	20	
Water	0	240 Cal
SNACK		
Coffee or tea	10	10 Cal
DINNER		
Cheeseburger (Day 30 Recipe - page 142)	320	
Lettuce and sliced tomato	20	
GF bun	180	
Steamed green beans	25	
Pickle spear	0	
Water	0	545 Cal
SNACK		
Coffee or tea	10	10 Cal
		1195 Cal

Day 31 1200 Calorie Meal Plan

BREAKFAST	Calories	Totals
Grapefruit (½)	75	
Scrambled egg	80	
GF bread - toasted (1 slice)	70	
Coffee	10	235 Cal
SNACK		
GF Yogurt (6 oz)	90	
Coffee or tea	10	100 Cal
LUNCH		
Ham (2 oz) with mustard on 2 slices GF bread	290	
Pickle spear	0	
Hot or iced tea	10	300 Cal
SNACK		
Fresh fruit in season (apple, plum, etc)	70	
Coffee or tea	10	80 Cal
DINNER		
Baked Sea Bass (Day 31 Recipe - page 143)	395	
Large tossed salad with 1½ Tbsp lite GF dressing	70	
Hot or iced tea	10	475 Cal
SNACK		
Coffee or tea	10	10 Cal
		1200 Cal

Day 32 1200 Calorie Meal Plan

BREAKFAST	Calories	Totals
Grapefruit (½)	75	
Glutino Honey Nut* (¾ cup) + ½ cup skim milk + ½ banana	215	
Coffee	10	300 Cal
* GF Cereal		
SNACK		
Coffee or tea	10	10 Cal
LUNCH		
GF Cottage cheese* (1 cup no fat)	140	
Tossed salad with 1½ Tbsp lite GF dressing	70	
GF bread (1 slice)	70	
Hot or iced tea	10	290 Cal
* Cabot No-Fat Cottage Cheese is gluten free		
SNACK		
Handful unsalted mixed nuts	100	
Coffee or tea	10	110 Cal
DINNER		
Turkey tenders & **veggies (Day 32 Recipe** -page144)	350	
Spinach (½ cup steamed & drizzled with 1 tsp	70	
Romaine lettuce, tomato slices & 1 Tbsp lite GF	45	
Water	0	465 Cal
SNACK		
GF Ginger-Snap Cookie	40	
Coffee or tea	10	50 Cal
		1210 Cal

Day 33 1200 Calorie Meal Plan

BREAKFAST	Calories	Totals
Cantaloupe (½ medium)	50	
Fried egg	80	
GF turkey bacon (1 slice)	35	
GF raisin bread - toasted (1 slice)	75	
Coffee	10	250 Cal
SNACK		
GF Yogurt (6 oz)	90	
Coffee or tea	10	100 Cal
LUNCH		
GF Soup (Appendix C - page 225)	150	
GF bread (1 slice)	70	
Lettuce and sliced tomato with 1 Tbsp lite GF	45	
Water	0	265 Cal
SNACK		
Coffee or tea	10	10 Cal
DINNER		
Frozen dinner (Day 33 Recipe - page 145)	340	
Large tossed salad with 1½ Tbsp lite GF dressing	70	
GF bread (1 slice)	70	
Fresh fruit in season (peach, plum, etc)	70	
Water	0	550 Cal
SNACK		
Coffee or tea	10	10 Cal
		1195 Cal

Day 34 1200 Calorie Meal Plan

BREAKFAST	Calories	Totals
Orange juice (½ cup)	50	
Rice Chex (1 cup) + ½ cup skim milk + ½ banana	195	
Coffee	10	255 Cal
SNACK		
Coffee or tea	10	10 Cal
LUNCH		
Roast beef (2 oz) sandwich (with lettuce)	300	
Hot or iced tea	10	310 Cal
SNACK		
Handful unsalted mixed nuts	100	
Coffee or tea	10	110 Cal
DINNER		
Pasta Rapini (Day 34 Recipe - page 147)	290	
Large tossed green salad with 1½ Tbsp lite GF	70	
GF bread (1 slice)	70	
Water	0	430 Cal
SNACK		
Fresh fruit in season (apple, peach, etc)	70	
Coffee or tea	10	80 Cal
		1195 Cal

Day 35 1200 Calorie Meal Plan

BREAKFAST	Calories	Totals
Cantaloupe (½ medium)	50	
GF Oatmeal (½ cup dry) + ½ cup skim milk + about 15 raisins	230	
Coffee	10	290 Cal
SNACK		
Fresh fruit in season (apple, peach, etc)	70	
Coffee or tea	10	80 Cal
LUNCH		
Grilled cheese sandwich* (2 slices GF light cheese)	270	
Pickle spear	0	
Hot or ice tea	10	280 Cal
* Sandwich has 2 slices GF bread		
SNACK		
Coffee or tea	10	10 Cal
DINNER		
Eat Out – Chicken dinner (Day 35 Recipe - page 148)		
Max allowable calories	530	530 Cal
SNACK		
Coffee or tea	10	10 Cal
		1200 Cal

Day 36 1200 Calorie Meal Plan

BREAKFAST	Calories	Totals
Cantaloupe (½ medium)	50	
Rice Krispies* (1 cup) + ½ cup skim milk + about 15 raisins	200	
Coffee	10	260 Cal
* Gluten free variety		
SNACK		
Fresh fruit in season (apple, pear, etc)	70	
Coffee or tea	10	80 Cal
LUNCH		
GF Soup (Appendix C - page 225)	140	
GF Turkey (1 oz) on 1 slice GF bread (½ sandwich)	120	
Water	0	260 Cal
SNACK		
Coffee or tea	10	10 Cal
DINNER		
Grilled Tilapia (Day 36 Recipe - page 150)	300	
Asparagus (6 spears)	25	
GF Wild rice* (½ cup – after cooking)	100	
Large tossed salad with 1½ Tbsp lite GF dressing	70	
Water	0	495 Cal
SNACK		
Popcorn Mini Bag	100	
Coffee or tea	10	110 Cal
* Rice is naturally gluten free.		1215 Cal

Day 37 1200 Calorie Meal Plan

BREAKFAST	Calories	Totals
Orange juice (½ cup)	50	
Soft-boiled egg	80	
GF bread - toasted (1 slice)	70	
Coffee	10	210 Cal
SNACK		
GF Yogurt (6 oz)	90	
Coffee or tea	10	100 Cal
LUNCH		
Salad (3 oz canned tuna*, 1 tsp Evoo, onions, celery)	175	
Lettuce & tomato wedges + GF bread (1 slice)	90	
Fresh fruit in season – (apple, pear, etc)	70	
Coffee or tea	10	345 Cal
SNACK		
Coffee or tea	10	10 Cal
DINNER		
Low-Cal Beef Stew (Day 37 Recipe - page 151)	365	
Large tossed salad with 1½ Tbsp lite GF dressing	70	
GF bread - (1 slice)	70	
Water with lemon wedge	10	515 Cal
SNACK		
Coffee or tea	10	10 Cal
* Chicken of the Sea & Bumble Bee are gluten free.		1190 Cal

Day 38 1200 Calorie Meal Plan

BREAKFAST	Calories	Totals
Cantaloupe (½ medium)	50	
Smoothie (Day 14 Recipe - page 124)	220	
Coffee	10	280 Cal
SNACK		
Coffee or tea	10	10 Cal
LUNCH		
GF Peanut butter (2 Tbsp) on 2 slices GF bread	330	
Skim milk (4 oz) need to add 45 Cal	45	375 Cal
SNACK		
Fresh fruit in season (apple, plum, etc)	70	
Coffee or tea	10	80 Cal
DINNER		
Pan-broiled lamb chop (Day 38 Recipe - page 152)	320	
Large tossed salad with 1½ Tbsp lite GF dressing	70	
Water	0	390 Cal
SNACK		
Coffee or tea	10	10 Cal
		1190 Cal

Day 39 1200 Calorie Meal Plan

BREAKFAST	Calories	Totals
Fresh sliced orange	75	
Cinnamon Chex (1 cup) + ½ cup skim milk + about	240	
Coffee	10	325 Cal
SNACK		
Fresh fruit in season (peach, plum, etc)	70	
Coffee or tea	10	80 Cal
LUNCH		
GF Cottage cheese (1 cup no fat)	140	
Large tossed salad with 1½ Tbsp lite GF dressing	70	
GF bread (1 slice)	70	
Hot or iced tea	10	290 Cal
SNACK		
Handful unsalted mixed nuts	100	
Coffee or tea	10	110 Cal
DINNER		
Chicken with veggies (Day 39 Recipe - page 153)	365	
Water with lemon wedge	10	375 Cal
SNACK		
Coffee or tea	10	10 Cal
		1190 Cal

Day 40 1200 Calorie Meal Plan

BREAKFAST	Calories	Totals
Orange juice (½ cup)	50	
Scrambled egg	80	
GF raisin bread - toasted (1 slice)	70	
Coffee	10	210 Cal
SNACK		
GF Yogurt (6 oz)	90	
Coffee or tea	10	100 Cal
LUNCH		
GF Soup (Appendix C - page 225)	160	
GF bread (1 slice)	70	
Water	0	230 Cal
SNACK		
Coffee or tea	10	10 Cal
DINNER		
Eat Out – Fish dinner (Day 40 Recipe - page 154)		
Max allowable calories	595	595 Cal
SNACK		
GF Cookie	60	
Coffee or tea	10	70 Cal
		1215 Cal

Day 41 1200 Calorie Meal Plan

BREAKFAST	Calories	Totals
Orange juice (½ cup)	50	
GF Oatmeal (½ cup dry) + ½ cup skim milk +about 15 raisins	230	
Coffee	10	290 Cal
SNACK		
Coffee or tea	10	10 Cal
LUNCH		
GF Turkey Hot Dog (page 221) w mustard & relish	100	
GF Hot-dog bun	150	
Diet soda (or water)	0	250 Cal
SNACK		
Handful unsalted mixed nuts	100	
Coffee or tea	10	110 Cal
DINNER		
Pasta e Fagioli (Day 41 Recipe - page 155)	300	
Large tossed salad with 1½ Tbsp lite GF dressing	70	
GF bread (1 slice)	70	
Water with lemon wedge	10	450 Cal
SNACK		
Skinny Cow Chocolate Truffle Bar (ice cream)	100	
Coffee or tea	10	110 Cal
* Skinny Cow ice cream products are gluten free.		1220 Cal

Day 42 1200 Calorie Meal Plan

BREAKFAST	Calories	Totals
Cantaloupe (½ medium)	50	
Rice Chex (1 cup) + ½ cup skim milk + ½ banana	195	
Coffee	10	255 Cal
SNACK		
Coffee or tea	10	10 Cal
LUNCH		
Grilled Swiss cheese sandwich* (2 slices GF light cheese)	270	
Pickle spear	0	
Hot or iced tea	10	320 Cal
* Sandwich has 2 slices GF bread.		
SNACK		
Fresh fruit in season (apple, peach, etc)	70	
Coffee or tea	10	80 Cal
DINNER		
Frozen dinner (Day 28 Recipe - page 139)	300	
Large tossed salad with 1½ Tbsp lite GF dressing	70	
Water with lemon wedge	10	380 Cal
SNACK		
GF Blueberry Muffin (Day 42 Recipe - page 156)	125	
Coffee or tea	10	135 Cal
		1180 Cal

Day 43 1200 Calorie Meal Plan

BREAKFAST	Calories	Totals
Fresh or frozen strawberries (½ cup)	25	
French toast (Day 3 Recipe - page 111)	310	
GF Lite Syrup (1 Tbsp)	30	
Coffee	10	375 Cal
SNACK		
GF Yogurt (6 oz)*	90	
Coffee or tea	10	100 Cal
LUNCH		
Salad (3 oz canned tuna, 1 tsp Evoo, onions, celery)	175	
Lettuce & tomato wedges	20	
GF bread (½ slice)	35	
Diet soda (or water)	0	230 Cal
SNACK		
Coffee or tea	10	10 Cal
DINNER		
Beef Kebob with veggies (Day 43 Recipe - page 157)	390	
Baked potato (medium)	100	
Water	0	490 Cal
SNACK		
Coffee or tea	10	10 Cal
* Such as Yoplait Light which is non-fat & gluten free.		1215 Cal

Day 44 1200 Calorie Meal Plan

BREAKFAST	Calories	Totals
Orange juice (½ cup)	50	
Rice Krispies (1 cup) + ½ cup skim milk + ½ banana	205	
Coffee	10	265 Cal
SNACK		
Fresh fruit in season (apple, peach, etc)	70	
Coffee or tea	10	80 Cal
LUNCH		
GF Soup (Appendix C - page 225)	90	
GF bread	70	
Hot or iced tea	10	170 Cal
SNACK		
Popcorn Mini Bag*	100	
Coffee or tea	10	110 Cal
DINNER		
Baked Haddock (Day 44 Recipe - page 158)	400	
Large tossed salad with 1½ Tbsp lite GF dressing	70	
Water with lemon wedge	10	480 Cal
SNACK		
Glutino Chocolate-Covered Pretzels**	75	
Coffee or tea	10	85 Cal
* Such as Orville Redenbacher's Smart Pop ** 5 pretzels		1190 Cal

Day 45 1200 Calorie Meal Plan

BREAKFAST	Calories	Totals
Cantaloupe (½ medium)	50	
Fried egg	80	
GF bread - toasted (1 slice)	70	
Coffee	10	210 Cal
SNACK		
GF Yogurt (6 oz)	90	
Coffee or tea	10	100 Cal
LUNCH		
GF Soup (Appendix C - page 225)	180	
Lettuce & tomato sandwich (Tbsp light GF mayo)*	170	
Water	0	360 Cal
* Sandwich with GF bread. See page 222 for GF mayo.		
SNACK		
Coffee or tea	10	10 Cal
DINNER		
Chicken Cacciatore (Day 45 Recipe - page 159)	310	
GF bread (1 slice)	70	
Water	0	380 Cal
SNACK		
GF Blueberry muffin	125	
Coffee or tea	10	135 Cal
		1195 Cal

Day 46 1200 Calorie Meal Plan

BREAKFAST	Calories	Totals
Grapefruit (½)	75	
Cinnamon Chex (1 cup) + ½ cup skim milk + ½ banana	255	
Coffee	10	300 Cal
SNACK		
Coffee or tea	10	10 Cal
LUNCH		
GF Cottage cheese (1 cup no fat)	140	
Large tossed salad with 1½ Tbsp lite dressing	70	
Hot or iced tea	10	220 Cal
SNACK		
Coffee or tea	10	10 Cal
DINNER		
Poached Cod (Day 46 Recipe - page 160)	275	
Grilled potatoes	100	
Grilled cherry tomatoes	45	
Spinach (½ cup) steamed with garlic & drizzled	50	
Water with lemon wedge	10	480 Cal
SNACK		
GF Blueberry muffin	125	
Coffee or tea	10	135 Cal
		1195 Cal

Day 47 1200 Calorie Meal Plan

BREAKFAST	Calories	Totals
Grapefruit (½)	75	
Scrambled egg	80	
GF bread - toasted (1 slice)	70	
Coffee	10	235 Cal
SNACK		
GF Yogurt (6 oz)	90	
Coffee or tea	10	100 Cal
LUNCH		
GF Soup (Appendix C - page 225)	80	
GF turkey breast (1 oz) on 1 slice GF bread (½ sandwich)	120	
Lettuce & tomato slices	20	220 Cal
SNACK		
Coffee or tea	10	10 Cal
DINNER		
Eat Out – Chinese food (Day 19 Recipe - page 129)		
Max allowable calories	640	640 Cal
* Order about 900 Cal. Take home ⅓ (about 300 Cal) for		
SNACK		
Coffee or tea	10	10 Cal
		1215 Cal

Day 48 1200 Calorie Meal Plan

BREAKFAST	Calories	Totals
Cantaloupe (½ medium)	50	
Smoothie (Day 14 Recipe - page 124)	220	
Coffee	10	280 Cal
SNACK		
Coffee or tea	10	10 Cal
LUNCH		
Left over Chinese food from Day 47	290	
Hot or iced tea	10	300 Cal
SNACK		
GF Ginger Snap Cookie	40	
Coffee or tea	10	50 Cal
DINNER		
Pasta Salad (Day 48 Recipe - page 162)	370	
GF bread (1 slice)	70	
Water	0	440 Cal
SNACK		
GF Blueberry muffin	125	
Coffee or tea	10	135 Cal
		1215 Cal

Day 49 1200 Calorie Meal Plan

BREAKFAST	Calories	Totals
Cantaloupe (½ medium)	50	
GF Oatmeal* (½ cup dry) + ½ cup skim milk + about 15 raisins	230	
Coffee	10	280 Cal
* See page 216.		
MORNING SNACK		
GF Ginger-Snap Cookie	40	
Coffee or tea	10	50 Cal
LUNCH		
GF Turkey breast (2 oz) on 2 slices GF bread	245	
Lettuce, tomato and 1 Tbsp light mayo	35	
Pickle spear	0	
Water with lemon wedge	10	290 Cal
SNACK		
Fresh fruit in season (apple, plum, etc)	70	
Coffee or tea	10	80 Cal
DINNER		
Frozen dinner (Day 21 Recipe - page 131)	300	
Large tossed salad with 1½ Tbsp lite GF dressing	70	
Water with lemon wedge	10	380 Cal
SNACK		
GF Blueberry muffin	125	
Coffee or tea	10	135 Cal
		1215 Cal

Day 50 1200 Calorie Meal Plan

BREAKFAST	Calories	Totals
Fresh or frozen strawberries (1 cup)	25	
French toast (Day 3 Recipe - page 111)	270	
GF Lite Syrup (1 Tbsp)	30	
Coffee	10	335 Cal
SNACK		
Coffee or tea	10	10 Cal
LUNCH		
GF Soup (Appendix C - page 225)	110	
BLT sandwich - lettuce & tomato*	270	
Pickle spear	0	
Hot or iced tea	10	390 Cal
* 2 slices GF turkey bacon & 1 Tbsp GF light mayo		
SNACK		
Coffee or tea	10	10 Cal
DINNER		
Pan-fried Sole (Day 50 Recipe - page 165)	325	
Large tossed salad with 1½ Tbsp lite GF dressing	70	
Water	0	395 Cal
SNACK		
GF Ginger-Snap Cookie	40	
Coffee or tea	10	50 Cal
		1190 Cal

Day 51 1200 Calorie Meal Plan

BREAKFAST	Calories	Totals
Cantaloupe (½ medium)	50	
Rice Chex (1 cup) + ½ cup skim milk + ½ banana	195	
Coffee	10	255 Cal
SNACK		
Coffee or tea	10	10 Cal
LUNCH		
Ham (2 oz) with mustard on 2 slices GF bread	290	
Pickle spear	0	
Hot or iced tea	10	300 Cal
SNACK		
Handful unsalted mixed nuts	100	
Coffee or tea	10	110 Cal
DINNER		
Beans and Greens Salad (Day 51 Recipe - page 166)	260	
GF bread (1 slice)	70	
Baked potato (medium)	100	
Water with lemon wedge	10	510 Cal
SNACK		
Coffee or tea	10	10 Cal
		1195 Cal

Day 52 1200 Calorie Meal Plan

BREAKFAST	Calories	Totals
Fresh orange sliced	75	
Soft-boiled egg	80	
GF bread - toasted (1 slice)	70	
Coffee	10	235 Cal
SNACK		
GF Yogurt (6 oz)	90	
Coffee or tea	10	100 Cal
LUNCH		
Salad – 3 oz canned salmon, 1 tsp Evoo, onions & celery	200	
Lettuce & tomato wedges	20	
Rye bread (1 slice)	70	
Water	0	290 Cal
SNACK		
Fresh fruit in season (apple, plum, etc)	70	
Coffee or tea	10	80 Cal
DINNER		
Chicken Piccata (Day 52 Recipe - page 167)	270	
Brown rice (½ cup – after cooking)	100	
Large tossed salad with 1½ Tbsp lite GF dressing	70	
Water	0	440 Cal
SNACK		
GF Ginger-Snap Cookie	40	
Coffee or tea	10	50 Cal
		1195 Cal

Day 53 1200 Calorie Meal Plan

BREAKFAST	Calories	Totals
Orange juice (½ cup)	50	
Rice Krispies (1 cup) + ½ cup skim milk + about 15 raisins	200	
Coffee	10	250 Cal
SNACK		
Fresh fruit in season (peach, plum, etc)	70	
Coffee or tea	10	80 Cal
LUNCH		
GF Cottage cheese (1 cup no fat)	140	
Tossed salad with 1½ Tbsp lite GF dressing	70	
Hot or iced tea	10	220 Cal
SNACK		
Handful unsalted mixed nuts	100	
Coffee or tea	10	110 Cal
DINNER		
Beef steak strips (Day 53 Recipe - page 168)	330	
Steamed spinach (½ cup)	25	
Baked potato (medium)	100	
GF bread (1 slice)	70	
Water with lemon wedge	10	535 Cal
SNACK		
Coffee or tea	10	10 Cal
		1205 Cal

Day 54 1200 Calorie Meal Plan

BREAKFAST	Calories	Totals
Cantaloupe (½ medium)	50	
Fried egg	80	
GF bread - toasted (1 slice)	70	
Coffee	10	210 Cal
SNACK		
GF Yogurt (6 oz)	90	
Coffee or tea	10	100 Cal
LUNCH		
GF Soup (Appendix C - page 225)	200	
GF bread (1 slice)	70	
Lettuce & tomato slices	20	
Water	0	300 Cal
SNACK		
GF Cookie	60	
Coffee or tea	10	70 Cal
DINNER		
Grilled scallops (Day 54 Recipe - page 169)	210	
Grilled polenta (Day 54)	125	
Mushroom-steamed green beans-red onion (Day 54)	45	
Grilled asparagus (Day 54)	10	
Large tossed salad with 1½ Tbsp lite GF dressing	70	
Water	0	460 Cal
SNACK		
Fresh fruit in season (apple, peach, etc)	70	
Coffee or tea	10	80 Cal
		1220 Cal

Day 55 1200 Calorie Meal Plan

BREAKFAST	Calories	Totals
Orange juice (½ cup)	50	
Cinnamon Chex (¾ cup) + ½ cup skim milk + ½ banana	215	
Coffee	10	275 Cal
SNACK		
Coffee or tea	10	10 Cal
LUNCH		
One servings left over Day 51 bean salad	270	
GF bread (1 slice)	80	
Lettuce & tomato slices	20	
Hot or iced tea	10	380 Cal
SNACK		
Coffee or tea	10	10 Cal
DINNER		
Hearty Vegetable Soup (Day 55 Recipe - page 170)	360	
Large tossed salad with 1½ Tbsp lite GF dressing	70	
GF bread (1 slice)	80	
Water	0	510 Cal
SNACK		
Coffee or tea	10	10 Cal
		1195 Cal

Day 56 1200 Calorie Meal Plan

BREAKFAST	Calories	Totals
Orange juice (½ cup)	50	
GF Oatmeal (½ cup dry) + ½ cup skim milk + about 15 raisins	230	
Coffee	10	290 Cal
SNACK		
Coffee or tea	10	10 Cal
LUNCH		
Roast beef (2 oz) sandwich on GF bread	295	
Lettuce & tomato slices	20	
Fresh fruit in season (peach, plum, etc)	70	
Water	0	385 Cal
SNACK		
Carrot sticks + ¼ cup no-fat cottage cheese & chives	55	
Coffee or tea	10	65 Cal
DINNER		
Frozen dinner (Day 28 Recipe - page 137)	300	
Large tossed salad with 1½ Tbsp lite GF dressing	70	
GF bread (1 slice)	70	
Water	0	440 Cal
SNACK		
Coffee or tea	10	10 Cal
		1200 Cal

Day 57 1200 Calorie Meal Plan

BREAKFAST	Calories	Totals
Cantaloupe (½ medium)	50	
Smoothie (Day 14 Recipe - page 124)	220	
Coffee	10	280 Cal
SNACK		
Coffee or tea	10	10 Cal
LUNCH		
Salad (3 oz canned tuna, 1 tsp Evoo, onions, celery)	175	
Lettuce & tomato wedges	20	
GF bread (1 slice)	70	
Fresh fruit in season (apple, pear, etc)	70	
Coffee or tea	10	345 Cal
SNACK		
Coffee or tea	10	10 Cal
DINNER		
Salmon w Mango Salsa (Day 57 Recipe - page 173)	460	
Large tossed salad with 1½ Tbsp lite GF dressing	70	
Water with lemon wedge	10	540 Cal
SNACK		
Coffee or tea	10	10 Cal
		1195 Cal

Day 58 1200 Calorie Meal Plan

BREAKFAST	Calories	Totals
Orange juice (½ cup)	50	
Corn Chex (1 cup) + ½ cup skim milk + ½ banana	215	
Coffee	10	275 Cal
SNACK		
Fresh fruit in season (apple, pear, etc)	70	
Coffee or tea	10	80 Cal
LUNCH		
GF Soup (Appendix C - page 225)	90	
GF bread (1 slice)	70	
Hot or iced tea	10	170 Cal
SNACK		
Coffee or tea	10	10 Cal
DINNER		
Pork chop with orange (Day 58 Recipe - page 174)	470	
Wild rice (¼ cup – after cooking)	50	
Asparagus (7 spear cooked & drained)	20	
Water with lemon wedge	10	550 Cal
SNACK		
GF Blueberry muffin	125	
Coffee or tea	10	135 Cal
		1220 Cal

Day 59 1200 Calorie Meal Plan

BREAKFAST	Calories	Totals
Grapefruit (½)	75	
Scrambled egg	80	
GF bread (1 slice)	70	
Coffee	10	235 Cal
SNACK		
GF Yogurt (6 oz)	90	
Coffee or tea	10	100 Cal
LUNCH		
GF Soup (Appendix C - page 225)	130	
Tomato slices with ¼ cup chopped fresh basil + 1	60	
GF bread (1 slice)	70	
Water	0	260 Cal
SNACK		
Coffee or tea	10	10 Cal
DINNER		
Eat Out – Fish dinner (Day 5 Recipe - page 113)		
Max allowable calories	595	595 Cal
SNACK		
Coffee or tea	10	10 Cal
		1210 Cal

Day 60 1200 Calorie Meal Plan

BREAKFAST	Calories	Totals
Grapefruit (½)	75	
Corn Chex (1 cup) + ½ cup skim milk + ½ banana	215	
Coffee	10	300 Cal
SNACK		
Coffee or tea	10	10 Cal
LUNCH		
GF Cottage cheese (1 cup no fat)	140	
Large tossed salad with 1½ Tbsp lite GF dressing	70	
Hot or iced tea	10	220 Cal
SNACK		
Handful unsalted mixed nuts	100	
Coffee or tea	10	110 Cal
DINNER		
Chicken Stew (Day 60 Recipe - page 176)	360	
Brown rice (½ cup – after cooking)	100	
GF bread (1 slice)	80	
Water with lemon wedge	10	550 Cal
SNACK		
Coffee or tea	10	10 Cal
		1200 Cal

Day 61 1200 Calorie Meal Plan

BREAKFAST	Calories	Totals
Orange juice (½ cup)	50	
Chocolate Chex (¾ cup) + ½ cup skim milk + ½ banana	225	
Coffee	10	285 Cal
SNACK		
Coffee or tea	10	10 Cal
LUNCH		
GF Soup (Appendix C - page 225)	110	
GF turkey breast (1 oz) on 1 slice GF bread	120	
Pickle spear	0	
Lettuce & tomato slices	20	
Water	0	250 Cal
SNACK		
Coffee or tea	10	10 Cal
DINNER		
Shrimp over Spaghetti (Day 61 Recipe - page 177)	450	
Large tossed salad with 1½ Tbsp lite GF dressing	70	
Water with lemon wedge	10	530 Cal
SNACK		
Popcorn Mini Bag	100	
Coffee or tea	10	110 Cal
		1195 Cal

Day 62 1200 Calorie Meal Plan

BREAKFAST	Calories	Totals
Fresh or frozen strawberries (½ cup)	25	
French toast (Day 3 Recipe - page 111)	310	
GF Lite Syrup (1 Tbsp)	30	
Coffee	10	375 Cal
SNACK		
GF Yogurt (6 oz)*	90	
Coffee or tea	10	100 Cal
LUNCH		
Salad (3 oz canned tuna, 1 tsp Evoo, onions, celery)	175	
Lettuce & tomato wedges	20	
GF bread (1 slice)	70	
Water	0	265 Cal
SNACK		
Coffee or tea	10	10 Cal
DINNER		
Beef Burgundy (Day 62 Recipe - page 178)	350	
Large tossed salad with 1½ Tbsp lite GF dressing	70	
Water with lemon wedge	10	430 Cal
SNACK		
Coffee or tea	10	10 Cal
* Such as Yoplait Light which is non-fat & gluten free.		1190 Cal

Day 63 1200 Calorie Meal Plan

BREAKFAST	Calories	Totals
Grapefruit (½)	75	
Scrambled egg	80	
GF bread - toasted (1 slice)	70	
Coffee	10	235 Cal
SNACK		
GF Yogurt (6 oz)	90	
Coffee or tea	10	100 Cal
LUNCH		
Ham (2 oz) with mustard on 2 slices GF bread	290	
Pickle spear	0	
Water	0	290 Cal
SNACK		
Coffee or tea	10	10 Cal
DINNER		
Chicken cutlet (Day 63 Recipe - page 179)	450	
One small baked potato	50	
Large tossed salad with 1½ Tbsp lite GF dressing*	70	
Water	0	570 Cal
* Day 63 recipe shows much of salad on dinner plate.		
SNACK		
Coffee or tea	10	10 Cal
		1215 Cal

Day 64 1200 Calorie Meal Plan

BREAKFAST	Calories	Totals
Grapefruit (½)	75	
Glutino Honey Nut (¾ cup) + ½ cup skim milk + ½ banana	215	
Coffee	10	300 Cal
SNACK		
Coffee or tea	10	10 Cal
LUNCH		
GF Cottage cheese (1 cup no fat)	140	
Tossed salad with 1½ Tbsp lite dressing	70	
Water	0	210 Cal
SNACK		
Coffee or tea	10	10 Cal
DINNER		
Personal-Size Meat Loaf (Day 64 Recipe - page 180)	410	
Brown rice (½ cup – after cooking)	100	
Green beans - steamed	30	
Water	0	540 Cal
SNACK		
GF Blueberry muffin	125	
Coffee or tea	10	135 Cal
		1205 Cal

Day 65 1200 Calorie Meal Plan

BREAKFAST	Calories	Totals
Cantaloupe (½ medium)	50	
Smoothie (Day 14 Recipe page 124)	220	
Coffee	10	280 Cal
SNACK		
Coffee or tea	10	10 Cal
LUNCH		
GF Soup (Appendix C - page 225)	130	
GF bread (1 slice)	70	
Coffee or tea	10	210 Cal
SNACK		
Fresh fruit in season (apple, plum, etc)	70	
Coffee or tea	10	80 Cal
DINNER		
Frozen dinner (Day 5 Recipe - page 113)	340	
Large tossed salad with 1½ Tbsp lite GF dressing	70	
GF bread (1 slice)	70	
Water with lemon wedge	10	490 Cal
SNACK		
Popcorn Mini Bag	100	
Coffee or tea	10	110 Cal
		1180 Cal

Day 66 1200 Calorie Meal Plan

BREAKFAST	Calories	Totals
Orange juice (½ cup)	50	
Corn Chex (1 cup) + ½ cup skim milk + ½ banana	215	
Coffee	10	275 Cal
SNACK		
Fresh fruit in season (apple, plum, etc)	70	
Coffee or tea	10	80 Cal
LUNCH		
Left over meat loaf (½ of Day 64 serving)	205	
GF bread (1 slice)	70	
Lettuce	10	
Water	0	285 Cal
SNACK		
Handful unsalted mixed nuts	100	
Coffee or tea	10	110 Cal
DINNER		
Pepper & Mushroom Pizza (Day 66 Recipe -page 183)	265	
Large tossed salad with 1½ Tbsp lite GF dressing	70	
Water with lemon wedge	10	345 Cal
SNACK		
Skinny Cow Chocolate Truffle Bar	100	
Coffee or tea	10	110 Cal
		1205 Cal

Day 67 1200 Calorie Meal Plan

BREAKFAST	Calories	Totals
Cantaloupe (½ medium)	50	
Corn Chex (1 cup) + ½ cup skim milk + about 15 raisins	200	
Coffee	10	260 Cal
SNACK		
Coffee or tea	10	10 Cal
LUNCH		
GF Soup (Appendix C - page 225)	70	
Grilled cheese sandwich* (2 slices GF light cheese)	270	
Lettuce and sliced tomato	20	
Pickle spear	0	
Water	0	360 Cal
SNACK		
Coffee or tea	10	10 Cal
DINNER		
Eat Out – Chicken dinner (Day 7 Recipe -page 116)		
Max allowable calories	530	530 Cal
SNACK		
Coffee or tea	10	10 Cal
		1180 Cal

Day 68 1200 Calorie Meal Plan

BREAKFAST	Calories	Totals
Orange juice (½ cup)	50	
Cream of Rice (1 packet) + ½ cup skim milk +	230	
Coffee	10	290 Cal
SNACK		
Coffee or tea	10	10 Cal
LUNCH		
GF Soup (Appendix C - page 225)	90	
Turkey (1 oz) on 1 slice GF bread (½ sandwich)	120	
Lettuce	5	
Water	0	215 Cal
SNACK		
Coffee or tea	10	10 Cal
DINNER		
Pork Medallions lime sauce (Day 68 Recipe -page 186)	450	
Green beans - steamed	25	
Large tossed salad with 1½ Tbsp lite GF dressing	70	
Water with lemon wedge	10	555 Cal
SNACK		
Popcorn Mini Bag	100	
Coffee or tea	10	110 Cal
		1190 Cal

Day 69 1200 Calorie Meal Plan

BREAKFAST	Calories	Totals
Orange juice (½ cup)	50	
Soft-boiled egg	80	
GF bread - toasted (1 slice)	70	
Coffee	10	210 Cal
SNACK		
GF Yogurt (6 oz)	90	
Coffee or tea	10	100 Cal
LUNCH		
Salad (3 oz canned tuna*, 1 tsp Evoo, onions, celery)	175	
Lettuce & tomato wedges + GF bread (1 slice)	90	
Fresh fruit in season – (apple, peach, etc)	70	
Coffee or tea	10	345 Cal
* Chicken of the Sea & Bumble Bee are GF.		
SNACK		
Coffee or tea	10	10 Cal
DINNER		
Healthy Chicken Salad (Day 69 Recipe - page 187)	330	
GF bread (1 slice)	70	
Water with lemon wedge	10	410 Cal
SNACK		
Handful unsalted mixed nuts	100	
Coffee or tea	10	110 Cal
		1185 Cal

Day 70 1200 Calorie Meal Plan

BREAKFAST	Calories	Totals
Orange juice (½ cup)	50	
Wild blueberry pancakes (Day 10 Recipe -page 120)	190	
GF Lite Syrup (1½ Tbsp)	45	
Coffee	10	295 Cal
SNACK		
Coffee or tea	10	10 Cal
LUNCH		
GF Peanut butter (2 Tbsp) on 2 slices of GF bread	330	
Skim milk (6 oz)	65	395 Cal
SNACK		
Fresh fruit in season (apple, peach, etc)	70	
Coffee or tea	10	80 Cal
DINNER		
Baked Cod (Day 70 Recipe - page 188)	230	
Brown rice (½ cup – after cooking)	100	
Green beans - steamed	25	
Zucchini, tomatoes & onion – steamed	45	
Water	0	400 Cal
SNACK		
Coffee or tea	10	10 Cal
		1190 Cal

Day 71 1200 Calorie Meal Plan

BREAKFAST	Calories	Totals
Fresh sliced orange	75	
Chocolate Chex (¾ cup) + ½ cup skim milk + ½ banana	225	
Coffee	10	310 Cal
SNACK		
Coffee or tea	10	10 Cal
LUNCH		
GF Cottage cheese* (1 cup no fat)	140	
Large tossed salad with 1½ Tbsp lite GF dressing	70	
GF bread (1 slice)	70	
Hot or iced tea	10	290 Cal
SNACK		
Fresh fruit in season (apple, peach, etc)	70	
Coffee or tea	10	80 Cal
DINNER		
Chicken Scaloppini (Day 71 Recipe - page 189)	260	
White Rice (½ cup – after cooking)	100	
Snow peas or green beans - steamed	25	
Water with lemon wedge	10	395 Cal
SNACK		
GF Blueberry muffin (Day 42 Recipe - page 156)	125	
Coffee or tea	10	135 Cal
		1220 Cal

Day 72 1200 Calorie Meal Plan

BREAKFAST	Calories	Totals
Grapefruit (½)	75	
Scrambled egg	80	
GF bread - toasted (1 slice)	70	
Coffee	10	235 Cal
SNACK		
GF Yogurt (6 oz)	90	
Coffee or tea	10	100 Cal
LUNCH		
GF Soup (Appendix C - page 225)	160	
GF bread (1 slice)	70	
Hot or iced tea	10	240 Cal
SNACK		
Coffee or tea	10	10 Cal
DINNER		
Eat Out – Fish dinner (Day 72 Recipe - page 190)		
Maximum allowable calories	595	595 Cal
SNACK		
Coffee or tea	10	10 Cal
		1190 Cal

Day 73 1200 Calorie Meal Plan

BREAKFAST	Calories	Totals
Orange juice (½ cup)	50	
Glutino Honey Nut (¾ cup) + ½ cup skim milk + ½ banana	215	
Coffee	10	275 Cal
SNACK		
Coffee or tea	10	10 Cal
LUNCH		
Turkey frank (2 oz) with mustard & relish	150	
Hot-dog bun	130	
Diet soda	0	280 Cal
SNACK		
Coffee or tea	10	10 Cal
DINNER		
Pasta Pomodoro (Day 73 Recipe - page 191)	420	
Large tossed salad with 1½ Tbsp lite GF dressing	70	
GF bread (1 slice)	70	
Water with lemon wedge	10	570 Cal
SNACK		
GF Ginger-Snap Cookie	40	
Coffee or tea	10	50 Cal
		1195 Cal

Day 74 1200 Calorie Meal Plan

BREAKFAST	Calories	Totals
Cantaloupe (½ medium)	50	
Rice Chex (1 cup) + ½ cup skim milk + ½ banana	195	
Coffee	10	255 Cal
SNACK		
Fresh fruit in season (peach, plum, etc)	70	
Coffee or tea	10	80 Cal
LUNCH		
Grilled cheese sandwich (2 slices GF light cheese)	270	
Pickle spear	0	
Hot or iced tea	10	290 Cal
SNACK		
GF Ginger-Snap Cookie	40	
Coffee or tea	10	50 Cal
DINNER		
Frozen dinner (Day 74 Recipe - page 192)	300	
Large tossed salad with 1½ Tbsp lite GF dressing	70	
Water with lemon wedge	10	380 Cal
SNACK		
GF Blueberry Muffin	125	
Coffee or tea	10	135 Cal
		1190 Cal

Day 75 1200 Calorie Meal Plan

BREAKFAST	Calories	Totals
Cantaloupe (½ medium)	50	
Smoothie (Day 14 Recipe - page 124)	220	
Coffee	10	280 Cal
SNACK		
Handful unsalted mixed nuts	100	
Coffee or tea	10	110 Cal
LUNCH		
Salad (3 oz canned tuna, 1 tsp Evoo, onions, celery)	175	
Lettuce & tomato wedges	20	
GF bread (1 slice)	70	
Coffee or tea	10	275 Cal
SNACK		
Coffee or tea	10	10 Cal
DINNER		
Szechuan Noodles & Pork (Day 75 Recipe - page 194)	440	
Large tossed salad with 1½ Tbsp lite GF dressing	70	
Water with lemon wedge	10	520 Cal
SNACK		
Coffee or tea	10	10 Cal
		1205 Cal

Day 76 1200 Calorie Meal Plan

BREAKFAST	Calories	Totals
Orange juice (½ cup)	50	
Rice Krispies (1 cup) + ½ cup skim milk + about 15 raisins	200	
Coffee	10	260 Cal
SNACK		
Fresh fruit in season (apple, peach, etc)	70	
Coffee or tea	10	80 Cal
LUNCH		
GF Soup (Appendix C - page 225)	90	
GF bread (1 slice)	80	
Hot or iced tea	10	180 Cal
SNACK		
GF Ginger-Snap Cookie	40	
Coffee or tea	10	50 Cal
DINNER		
Grilled Sea Scallops (Day 76 Recipe page 195)	200	
Corn on the cob – one ear	100	
Tomato slices drizzled with Evoo	60	
Large tossed salad with 1½ Tbsp lite GF dressing	70	
GF bread (1 slice)	80	
Water with lemon wedge	10	520 Cal
SNACK		
Popcorn Mini Bag	100	
Coffee or tea	10	110 Cal
		1200 Cal

Day 77 1200 Calorie Meal Plan

BREAKFAST	Calories	Totals
Cantaloupe (½ medium)	50	
Fried egg	80	
GF raisin bread - toasted (1 slice)	70	
Coffee	10	210 Cal
SNACK		
GF Yogurt (6 oz)	90	
Coffee or tea	10	100 Cal
LUNCH		
GF Soup (Appendix C - page 225)	150	
Lettuce & tomato sandwich (Tbsp light GF mayo)	180	
Cucumber slices and carrots & celery sticks	15	
Hot or iced tea	10	355 Cal
* Sandwich made with GF bread		
SNACK		
Coffee or tea	10	10 Cal
DINNER		
Chicken w Peppers & Rice (Day 77 Recipe page 196)	290	
Large tossed salad with 1½ Tbsp lite GF dressing	70	
GF bread (1 slice)	70	
Fresh fruit in season (apple, peach, etc)	70	
Water with lemon wedge	10	510 Cal
SNACK		
Coffee or tea	10	10 Cal
		1195 Cal

Day 78 1200 Calorie Meal Plan

BREAKFAST	Calories	Totals
Grapefruit (½)	75	
Cinnamon Chex (1 cup) + ½ cup skim milk + ½ banana	255	
Coffee	10	340 Cal
SNACK		
Coffee or tea	10	10 Cal
LUNCH		
Cottage cheese (1 cup no fat)	140	
Large tossed salad with 1½ Tbsp lite GF dressing	70	
GF bread	70	
Hot or iced tea	10	290 Cal
SNACK		
Coffee or tea	10	10 Cal
DINNER		
Trout w Lemon Capers (Day 78 Recipe - page 197)	340	
Wild rice (½ cup – after cooking)	100	
Green beans (steamed)	30	
Sautéed cherry tomatoes (Day 25 Recipe - page 136)	60	
Water with lemon wedge	10	540 Cal
SNACK		
Coffee or tea	10	10 Cal
		1200 Cal

Day 79 1200 Calorie Meal Plan

BREAKFAST	Calories	Totals
Grapefruit (½)	75	
Scrambled egg	80	
GF bread - toasted (1 slice)	70	
Coffee	10	235 Cal
SNACK		
GF Yogurt (6 oz)	90	
Coffee or tea	10	100 Cal
LUNCH		
GF Soup (Appendix C - page 225)	140	
GF bead (1 slice)	70	
Water	0	210 Cal
SNACK		
Coffee or tea	10	10 Cal
DINNER		
Eat Out – Chinese food (Day 79 Recipe - page 198)		
Max allowable calories	640	640 Cal
* Order about 900 Cal. Take home ⅓ for lunch on Day 80.		
SNACK		
Coffee or tea	10	10 Cal
		1205 Cal

Day 80 1200 Calorie Meal Plan

BREAKFAST	Calories	Totals
Tomato juice (½ cup)	20	
GF Oatmeal (½ cup dry) + ½ cup skim milk +about 15 raisins	230	
Coffee	10	260 Cal
SNACK		
Coffee or tea	10	10 Cal
LUNCH		
Left over Chinese food from Day 79	290	
Coffee or tea	10	300 Cal
SNACK		
Coffee or tea	10	10 Cal
DINNER		
Vegetable Chili (Day 80 Recipe - page 199)	360	
Brown rice (½ cup – after cooking)	100	
Large tossed salad with 1½ Tbsp lite GF dressing	70	
GF bread (1 slice)	70	
Water with lemon wedge	10	610 Cal
SNACK		
Coffee or tea	10	10 Cal
		1200 Cal

Day 81 1200 Calorie Meal Plan

BREAKFAST	Calories	Totals
Cantaloupe (½ medium)	50	
Rice Chex (1 cup) + ½ cup skim milk + ½ banana	195	
Coffee	10	255 Cal
SNACK		
Handful unsalted mixed nuts	100	
Coffee or tea	10	110 Cal
LUNCH		
Turkey breast (2 oz) sandwich*	245	
Lettuce, tomato and Tbsp light mayo	35	
Pickle spear	0	
Water	0	280 Cal
* Sandwich made with GF bread		
SNACK		
GF Yogurt (6 oz)**	90	
Coffee or tea	10	100 Cal
DINNER		
Frozen dinner (Day 81 Recipe - page 200)	300	
Large tossed salad with 1½ Tbsp lite GF dressing	70	
GF bread (1 slice)	70	
Water with lemon wedge	10	450 Cal
SNACK		
Coffee or tea	10	10 Cal
** Such as Yoplait Light which is non-fat & gluten free.		1205 Cal

Day 82 1200 Calorie Meal Plan

BREAKFAST	Calories	Totals
Fresh or frozen strawberries (1 cup)	25	
French toast (Day 3 Recipe - page 111)	270	
GF Lite Syrup (1 Tbsp)	30	
Coffee	10	335 Cal
SNACK		
Coffee or tea	10	10 Cal
LUNCH		
GF Soup (Appendix C - page 225)	100	
BLT sandwich - lettuce & tomato*	270	
Pickle spear	0	
Hot or ice tea	10	380 Cal
* 2 slices GF turkey bacon & 1 Tbsp GF light mayo		
SNACK		
Coffee or tea	10	10 Cal
DINNER		
Chinese Chicken Salad (Day 82 Recipe - page 202)	440	
Hot or iced tea	10	450 Cal
SNACK		
Coffee or tea	10	10 Cal
		1195 Cal

Day 83 1200 Calorie Meal Plan

BREAKFAST	Calories	Totals
Cantaloupe (½ medium)	50	
Rice Krispies (1 cup) + ½ cup skim milk + about 15 raisins	200	
Coffee	10	260 Cal
SNACK		
Fresh fruit in season (apple, peach, etc)	70	
Coffee or tea	10	80 Cal
LUNCH		
Ham (2 oz) with mustard on 2 slices GF bread	290	
Pickle spear	0	
Diet coke (or water)	0	290 Cal
SNACK		
Popcorn Mini Bag	100	
Coffee or tea	10	110 Cal
DINNER		
Lentil Soup (Day 83 Recipe - page 203)	260	
Large tossed salad with 1½ Tbsp lite GF dressing	70	
GF bread (1 slice)	70	
Water	0	400 Cal
SNACK		
GF Ginger-Snap Cookie	40	
Coffee or tea	10	50 Cal
		1200 Cal

Day 84 1200 Calorie Meal Plan

BREAKFAST	Calories	Totals
Fresh orange sliced	75	
Soft-boiled egg	80	
GF bread - toasted (1 slice)	70	
Coffee	10	235 Cal
SNACK		
GF Yogurt (6 oz)	90	
Coffee or tea	10	100 Cal
LUNCH		
Salad – 3 oz canned salmon, 1 tsp Evoo, onions & celery	200	
Lettuce & tomato wedges	20	
GF bread (1 slice)	70	
Coffee or tea	10	300 Cal
SNACK		
Coffee or tea	10	10 Cal
DINNER		
Turkey Burger (Day 84 Recipe - page 204)	360	
Green beans or asparagus - steamed	25	
Pickle spear	0	
Large tossed salad with 1½ Tbsp lite GF dressing	70	
Water with lemon wedge	10	465 Cal
SNACK		
Handful unsalted mixed nuts	100	
Coffee or tea	10	110 Cal
		1220 Cal

Day 85 1200 Calorie Meal Plan

BREAKFAST	Calories	Totals
Grapefruit (½)	75	
Cinnamon Chex (¾ cup) + ½ cup skim milk + ½ banana	215	
Coffee	10	300 Cal
SNACK		
Coffee or tea	10	10 Cal
LUNCH		
Cottage cheese (1 cup non fat)	140	
Large tossed salad with 1½ Tbsp lite GF dressing	70	
GF bread (1 slice)	70	
Coffee or tea	10	290 Cal
SNACK		
Fresh fruit in season (apple, plum, etc)	70	
Coffee or tea	10	80 Cal
DINNER		
Meat Loaf (Day 85 Recipe - page 205)	290	
One-half acorn squash (baked with ½ tsp maple syrup*)	90	
Spinach (½ cup steamed & drizzled with 1 tsp Evoo)	70	
GF bread (1 slice)	70	
Water	0	520 Cal
* Pure maple syrup is naturally gluten free		
SNACK		
Coffee or tea	10	10 Cal
		1210 Cal

Day 86 1200 Calorie Meal Plan

BREAKFAST	Calories	Totals
Cantaloupe (½ medium)	50	
Fried egg	80	
GF bread - toasted (1 slice)	70	
Coffee	10	210 Cal
SNACK		
GF Yogurt (6 oz)	90	
Coffee or tea	10	100 Cal
LUNCH		
GF Soup (Appendix C - page 225)	200	
GF bread (1 slice)	70	
Lettuce & tomato slices	20	
Hot or ice tea	10	300 Cal
SNACK		
Coffee or tea	10	10 Cal
DINNER		
Tuna & Bean Salad (Day 86 Recipe - page 206)	355	
GF bread (1 slice)	70	
Water with lemon wedge	10	435 Cal
SNACK		
Blueberry muffin	125	
Coffee or tea	10	135 Cal
		1190 Cal

Day 87 1200 Calorie Meal Plan

BREAKFAST	Calories	Totals
Cantaloupe (½ medium)	50	
Smoothie (Day 14 Recipe - page 124)	220	
Coffee	10	280 Cal
SNACK		
Fresh fruit in season (peach, plum, etc)	70	
Coffee or tea	10	80 Cal
LUNCH		
Leftover meat loaf (½ Day 85 serving size)	145	
GF bread (1 slice)	70	
Lettuce & tomato slices	20	
Water	0	235 Cal
SNACK		
Celery sticks + ¼ cup no-fat cottage cheese & chives	60	
Coffee or tea	10	70 Cal
DINNER		
Pasta Primavera (Day 87 Recipe - page 207)	460	
Large tossed salad with 1½ Tbsp lite GF dressing	70	
Water	0	530 Cal
SNACK		
Coffee or tea	10	10 Cal
		1205 Cal

Day 88 1200 Calorie Meal Plan

BREAKFAST	Calories	Totals
Tomato juice (½ cup)	20	
GF Oatmeal (½ cup dry) + ½ cup skim milk +about 15 raisins	230	
Coffee	10	260 Cal
SNACK		
Fresh fruit in season (peach, plum, etc)	70	
Coffee or tea	10	80 Cal
LUNCH		
Roast beef (2 oz) sandwich on GF bread	295	
Lettuce	0	
Hot or iced tea	10	315 Cal
SNACK		
Handful unsalted mixed nuts	100	
Coffee or tea	10	110 Cal
DINNER		
Frozen dinner (Day 88 Recipe - page 208)	300	
Large tossed salad with 1½ Tbsp lite GF dressing	70	
GF bread (1 slice)	70	
Water	0	440 Cal
SNACK		
Coffee or tea	10	10 Cal
		1215 Cal

Day 89 1200 Calorie Meal Plan

BREAKFAST	Calories	Totals
Orange juice (½ cup)	50	
Wild blueberry pancakes (Day 10 Recipe - page 120)	190	
GF Lite Syrup (1½ Tbsp)	45	
Coffee	10	295 Cal
SNACK		
GF Yogurt (6 oz)	90	
Coffee or tea	10	100 Cal
LUNCH		
Salad (3 oz canned tuna, 1 tsp Evoo, onions, celery)	175	
Lettuce & tomato wedges	20	
GF bread (1 slice)	70	
Water	0	265 Cal
SNACK		
Fresh fruit in season (apple, pear, etc)	70	
Coffee or tea	10	80 Cal
DINNER		
Fish stew (Day 89 Recipe - page 210)	300	
Large tossed salad with 1½ Tbsp lite GF dressing	70	
GF bread (1 slice)	70	
Water with lemon wedge	10	450 Cal
SNACK		
Coffee or tea	10	10 Cal
		1200 Cal

Day 90 1200 Calorie Meal Plan

BREAKFAST	Calories	Totals
Fresh orange sliced	75	
Rice Chex (1 cup) + ½ cup skim milk + ½ banana	195	
Coffee	10	280 Cal
SNACK		
Coffee or tea	10	10 Cal
LUNCH		
GF Soup (Appendix C - page 225)	120	
GF bread (1 slice)	70	
Raw zucchini slices, celery & carrot sticks	20	
Hot or iced tea	10	220 Cal
SNACK		
Coffee or tea	10	10 Cal
DINNER		
Veal w Mushrooms & Tomato (Day 90 Recipe -page 211)	520	
GF bread (1 slice)	70	
Water with lemon wedge	10	600 Cal
SNACK		
Fresh fruit in season (apple, plum, etc)	70	
Coffee or tea	10	80 Cal
		1200 Cal

Recipes & Diet Tips

Day 1- Recipe

<u>Chicken with Peppers & Onions</u>

4 boneless and skinless chicken breasts (about 5 oz each)

Coat the chicken breasts in a bottled GF barbeque sauce (page 217). Prepare medium-hot fire on well-oiled grill. Place breasts on grill, turning them every 4 minutes, for 10 to 12 minutes, or until done. (To check if breasts are done, the meat should be moist and white with no sign of pink when you cut into the breast.) Salt and pepper to taste.

2 medium red peppers, sliced
1 medium onion, sliced

Place peppers and onions in pan with 2 tablespoons fat-free gluten-free chicken stock (page 223). Sauté until stock is reduced. Spray pan lightly with non-stick cooking oil (page 222) and cook another 2 minutes. Salt and pepper to taste.

<u>Serves 4</u>. About 250 Calories per serving (for chicken only).

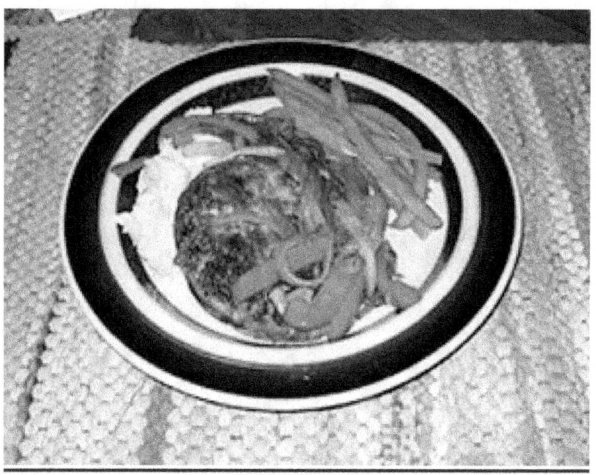

<u>Diet Tip of the Day:</u> Weight Loss – take it one step, one meal, one workout, one day at a time. Just think of where you'll be in 90 days!

Day 2 - Recipe

Baked Herb-Crusted Cod

4   cod fish fillets (4 to 5 ounces each)
2   tablespoons all-purpose GF free flour (page 215)
2   tablespoons GF cornmeal
2   tablespoons minced fresh herbs
2   teaspoons lemon juice

Sprinkle cod with lemon juice. Mix flour, cornmeal and herbs and dust the cod with the cornmeal-herb mixture. Bake in oven at 375 °F for 10 minutes. Add salt and black pepper to taste.

Serves 4. One serving is about 230 Calories (for cod only).

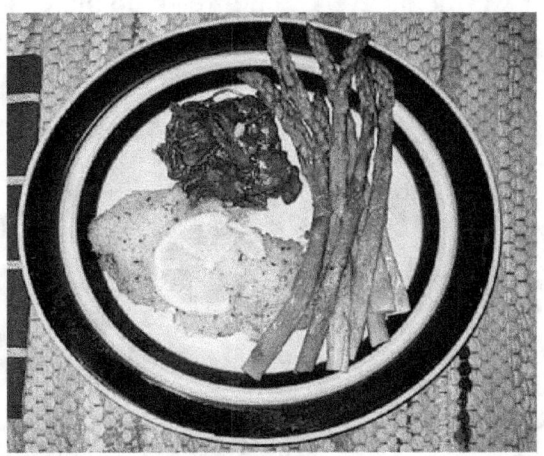

Diet Tip of the Day:. A **reducing diet is best supervised by a physician**. This is especially true when a great deal of weight needs to be lost, or if you have an ailment or a history of medical problems.

Day 3 - Recipe

French-Toast

    6 slices GF bread (page 216)*
    2 eggs
    ⅓ cup skim milk
    1 teaspoon vanilla
    A dash of cinnamon

In a medium bowl, beat together eggs and skim milk. Add vanilla and cinnamon. Saturate bread slices in egg mixture. In a non-stick skillet coated with cooking oil, cook bread slices until both sides are golden brown. If desired, dust lightly with confectionary sugar. Serve hot or keep in an oven or warmer at 200 ºF until ready to plate.
Serves 2. Three slices of French toast per serving. Each serving is 310 Calories.

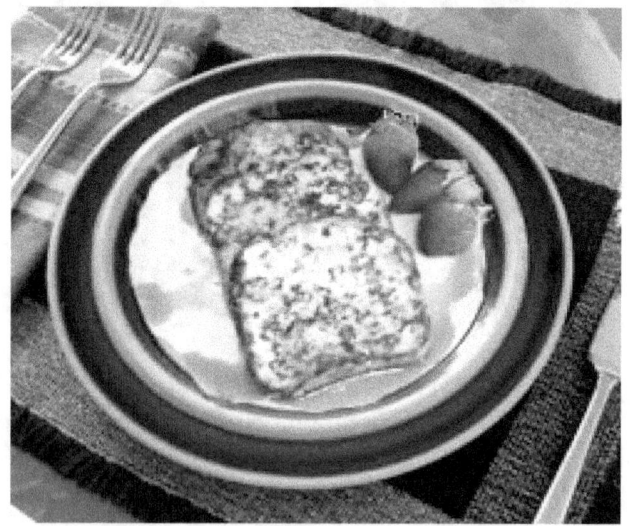

Diet Tip of the Day: "Eat Slowly" This is especially vital when you are trying to lose weight. If you are someone who eats fast, who finishes before everyone else at the table, you are not giving yourself a chance to feel full. While everyone else is still eating, you either sit there and pick, or you have seconds, taking in extra calories you could avoid if you would just slow down.

* We prepared this dish using Udi's gluten-free whole grain bread. Delicious!

Day 4 - Recipe

Carrie's Low-Cal Meat Loaf

½ pound ground white meat turkey
½ pound ground beef (about 90% lean)
1 large egg
½ cup skim milk
¼ cup GF bread crumbs (page 216)
¼ cup ketchup
¼ cup chopped carrots
¼ cup chopped onion

In a medium bowl, combine all ingredients. Add salt and pepper to taste. Mix until blended and form into a loaf. Place loaf into oven preheated to 350 °F. Bake until an instant-read thermometer inserted in the center of the loaf reads 160 °F. This should take about one hour.

Shown below is meat loaf, acorn squash (baked with 1 teaspoon of pure maple syrup). Also shown is steamed spinach drizzled with extra-virgin olive oil.

Serves 5. About 290 Calories per serving (for meat loaf only). Note: reserve half a serving of the meat loaf which is to be eaten for lunch on Day 6.

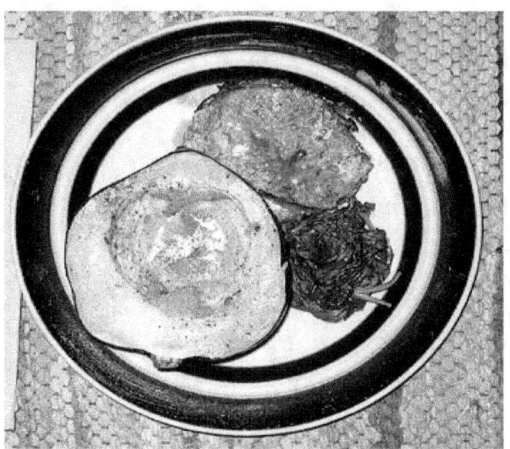

Diet Tip of the Day: **Buy a pedometer** and start walking. For the average person 2100 steps amounts to walking about one mile. A Harvard study has shown that 8000 to 10,000 step per day promote weight loss.

Day 5 - Recipe

<u>Frozen Dinner</u>

No recipe today. No cooking today. It's your day off! At this writing, Amy's and Artisan Bistro offer quite a few gluten-free frozen entrees. Smart Ones only makes two gluten-free entrees. Glutino also makes two gluten-free frozen entrees, but each contain 400 Calories, and are not included in the following list.

- Amy's Quinoa, Black Beans, Butternut Squash & Chard (**240 Cal**)
- Amy's Black Bean & Cheese Enchilada (**240 Cal**)
- Amy's Mushroom Risotto Bowl (**240 Cal**)
- Amy's Sweet & Sour Asian Noodle Bowl (**250 Cal**)
- Amy's Vegetable Parmesan Bowl (**260 Cal**)
- Amy's Brown Rice & Veggies Bowl – Light in Sodium (**260 Cal**)
- Amy's Brown Rice, Black-eyed Peas & Veggies Bowl (**290 Cal**)
- Amy's Teriyaki Bowl (**290 Cal**)
- Amy's Asian Noodle Stir Fry (**300 Cal**)
- Amy's Vegetable Lasagna (**300 Cal**)
- Amy's Thai Stir-Fry (**310 Cal**)
- Amy's Tofu Scramble (**320 Cal**)

- Artisan Bistro Wild Alaskan Salmon (**200 Cal**)
- Artisan Bistro Chicken Parmesan Bake (**200 Cal**)
- Artisan Bistro Turkey Cheddar Bake (**240 Cal**)
- Artisan Bistro Wild Alaskan Salmon Bake (**240 Cal**)
- Artisan Bistro Thai Style Yellow Curry with Chicken (**240 Cal**)
- Artisan Bistro Cheddar Beef Bake (**250 Cal**)
- Artisan Bistro Sesame Ginger with Salmon (**270 Cal**)
- Artisan Bistro Coconut Lemongrass with Chicken (**270 Cal**)
- Artisan Bistro Spiced Chicken Morocco (**270 Cal**)
- Artisan Bistro Albacore Tuna Bake (**280 Cal**)
- Artisan Bistro Thai Style Red Curry with Beef (**280 Cal**)
- Artisan Bistro Chicken Citron (**280 Cal**)
- Artisan Bistro Wild Alaskan Salmon with Pesto (**310 Cal**)
- Artisan Bistro Savory Turkey (**330 Cal**)
- Artisan Bistro Southwest Style Beef (**330 Cal**)
  - Artisan Bistro Ginger Chicken (**350 Cal**)
  - Artisan Bistro Beef with Mushroom Sauce (**350 Cal**)
  - Artisan Bistro Wild Alaskan Salmon Cake (**370 Cal**)

- Smart Ones Lemon Herb Chicken Piccata (**250 Cal**)
- Smart Ones Santa Fe Style Rice & Beans (**290 Cal**)

That's it. There are just not many low-calorie frozen GF entrees currently in stores. But more food manufacturers are getting on the GF band wagon, so check your local supermarket for the latest gluten-free frozen entrees. Also note that **340 Calories are allocated for this meal**. But almost all of the above have less than 340 Calories. Use the excess calories anyway you wish. Splurge on extra dessert or save the calories for another day! And please read the important **Frozen-Food Safety Warning** in **Appendix D** - page 226.

<u>Diet Tip of the Day:</u>   **Take a daily multi-vitamin/mineral supplement.** This is important when you're on a reducing diet – as a kind of insurance policy.

Day 6 - Recipe

Margherita Pizza

In the original 90-Day Smart Diet we featured a pizza recipe used by Gail Johnson's Italian grandmother. From feedback, our readers thought it was absolutely delicious - they loved it. We tried hard to make the pizza gluten free but just couldn't get the same crust and taste. After testing several commercially available brands of gluten-free pizza crust and finally settled on the following recipe (which makes two 9-inch pizzas):

    1   medium onion, minced & 1 clove of garlic, minced
    ¼   teaspoon dry oregano & ⅓.cup fresh basil leaves, torn
    3   oz part-skim mozzarella cheese, shredded
    2½ cups canned whole peeled tomatoes
    1   tablespoon extra-virgin olive oil, divided
    2   9-inch diameter GF pizza crust*

Tomato Sauce: Over medium high heat, sauté minced onion in two teaspoons of olive oil. Then stir in garlic, oregano, salt and pepper and ¼ teaspoon crushed red pepper (optional).. Add tomatoes including most of the juice in the can, crushing them as you put them in pan. Add ½ cup of water and simmer until sauce is reduced by one-half.

Brush one side of pizza crust with about a teaspoon of olive oil. Spread tomato sauce over crust and sprinkle shredded mozzarella cheese on top. Place pizza on the lower rack of an oven preheated to 375°F. Cook approximately 15 minutes or until cheese melts and bottom of pizza crust is brown. Sprinkle with fresh basil leaves. Cut and serve.

Serves 4. 230 Calories per serving. One full pizza shown below but a serving is half of a pizza.

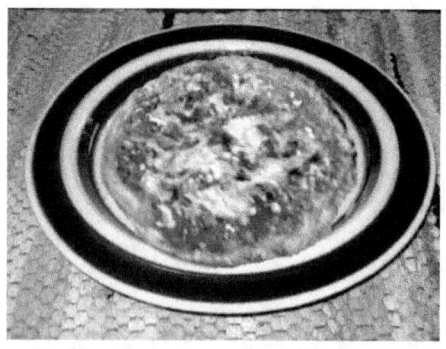

* We used Udi's GF Pizza Crust - 8 oz pkg which contains two 9-inch pizza crusts.

Day 7 - Recipe

Chicken Dinner - Out

No recipe today. No cooking today. Today you eat at a restaurant. But when you are on a gluten-free reducing diet, eating in a restaurant can be a double challenge. First, most restaurant portions are huge, easily totaling more than 1000 Calories, and then many restaurants do not offer gluten-free menu selections. On the *90-Day Gluten-Free Smart Diet*, a dinner type (i.e., fish, chicken, etc) and a calorie target are specified. For example Day 7 of the 1,200 Calorie diet calls for a chicken dinner and allows you 530 Calories for appetizer, soup, main course and dessert. Follow these tips to make sure your dinning experience is low calorie, gluten-free and pleasant.

Make sure you choose a restaurant where gluten-free food is available and where you have a fighting chance to achieve your calorie goal. Before you out go read the menu online and reduce your food choices so you can have more focused questions for the staff. You are more likely to get a safe meal if you call the restaurant before you go to let them know of your gluten-free needs. And call during a slow time so you can have the host's complete attention.

In the restaurant, to ensure you are served a gluten-free meal, it is important to communicate your need to eat 100 percent gluten-free assertively but amiably. Try to speak directly to the chef or manager. Otherwise, ask your server what is in the food and how it is prepared. Menu descriptions do not always list every ingredient. Inquire how gluten-free grains such as rice and risottos are cooked. Sometimes they are cooked in broth which may contain gluten. Confirm that separate, clean utensils and equipment will be used to prepare your meal.

Order something simple, such as skinless white meat broiled chicken breast with steamed vegetables and brown rice. Tell the waiter you want no sauce, no gravy, nothing added. Then, knowing your calorie objective, and that most fish and chicken are about 50 Calories per ounce, most steamed vegetable servings average approximately 50 Calories per cup, and rice is about 100 Calories per ½ cup, decide how much to eat – and take the remainder home. And consider bringing your own gluten-free salad dressing to the restaurant. If fresh fruit is not an option, pass on dessert and have the evening snack specified in the *90-Day Gluten-Free Smart Diet* meal plan for that day.

In a restaurant, most nutritionists recommend you eat the low-calorie items on your plate first. Start with the salad, soup and veggies. By the time you get to the chicken and starches you will hopefully be full enough to be content with smaller portions of the higher-calorie choices. (Incidentally, feel free to substitute skinless white meat turkey for chicken.)

We know that some dieticians advise their dieting clients not to eat out. They believe eating at home is safer. But our thought is you have to eat out eventually so why not learn how while your resolve is high?

Diet Tip of the Day: When you are on a diet and eating in a restaurant, a good rule of thumb is to **eat half of your entrée and bring the remainder home**.

Day 8 - Recipe

Baked Salmon with Salsa

This is a simple, straight-forward recipe. The advantage of a simple recipe is there are no hidden calories.

    4   5 oz salmon fillets
    6   tablespoons bottled salsa*

Brown salmon fillets in non-stick pan and then place them in a baking dish. Cook fillets in an oven preheated to 350 °F for about 10 minutes. Plate the salmon. Stir bottled tomato-pepper salsa and spoon it over the salmon.

Serves 4. One salmon fillet is about 215 Calories.

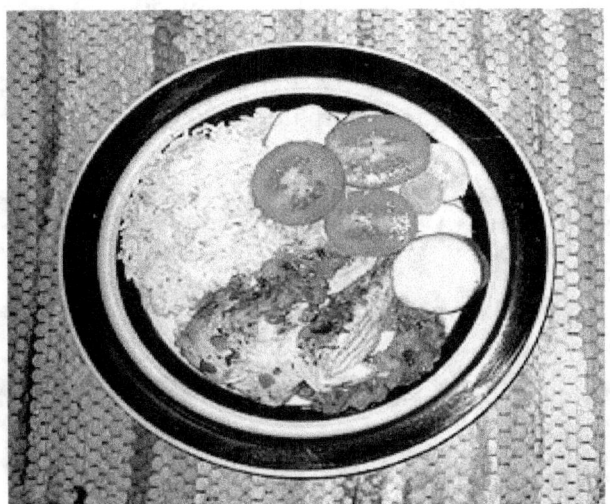

* We used Ortega's Garden Vegetable gluten-free salsa. See page 217 for other gluten-free salsas.

Diet Tip of the Day: Hunger is your body's way of telling you that you need calories. But **when you're done eating, you should feel better – satisfied but not stuffed**.

Day 9 - Recipe

Veggie Burger

Vegetable-based burgers can be purchased at your local supermarket. Patties of a veggie burger are made from either vegetables, soy, nuts, mushrooms, textured vegetable protein, dairy, or a combination of these foods.

Amy's makes two GF veggie burgers and Dr Paeger's makes one gluten free. Amy's GF Bistro Veggie Burger is made with organic, brown rice, pinto beans, plenty of mushrooms and barbeque sauce (110 Calories per patty). Amy's GF Sonoma Veggie Burger is made with organic vegetables, mushrooms and quinoa (140 Calories per patty). Dr Praeger's GF California Veggie Burger is made with many organic vegetables (110 Calories per patty).

Amy's Bistro Veggie Burger patty shown below plus a slice of light GF cheese amounts to approximately 180 Calories. The GF bun (page 216) increases the total to 360 Calories.

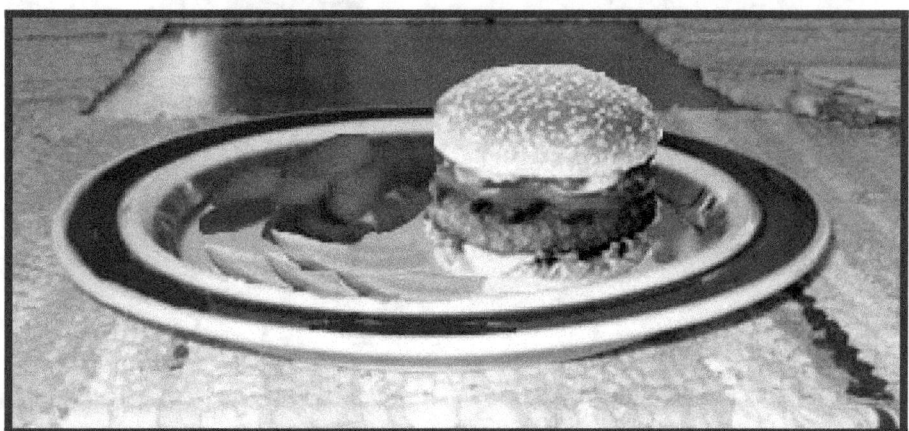

Photo shows seeded roll but most of the recommended GF burger rolls have no seeds.

Diet Tip of the Day: **Drink lots of water** – about 8 glasses per day when you're trying to lose weight. Add a slice of lemon to make it more interesting. Often, when you think you're hungry, you are just thirsty. So, next time you crave a snack, drink some water first and see if that does it for you.

Day 10 - Recipe

<u>Wild Blueberry Pancakes</u>

This recipe makes a relatively low calorie, wholesome batch of delicious gluten-free wild blueberry buttermilk pancakes.

    1½ cups gluten-free pancake mix (page 215)
    1 cup buttermilk
    1 egg
    1 tablespoon vegetable oil

Stir ingredients until blended. Add ¾ cup fresh of frozen blueberries and gently stir. Let batter stand about 15 minutes for fluffier pancakes. Using medium heat, preheat a non-stick skillet coated with cooking spray. Pour slightly less than ¼ cup of batter onto skillet per pancake. Cook slowly until bubbles break on surface of pancake. Turn and cook until other side is golden brown.

Makes 8 pancakes about 4-inches in diameter. Pictured below are two gluten-free blueberry pancakes with two slices of turkey bacon. **Serves 4**. Two pancakes per serving. Each pancake is about 105 Calories

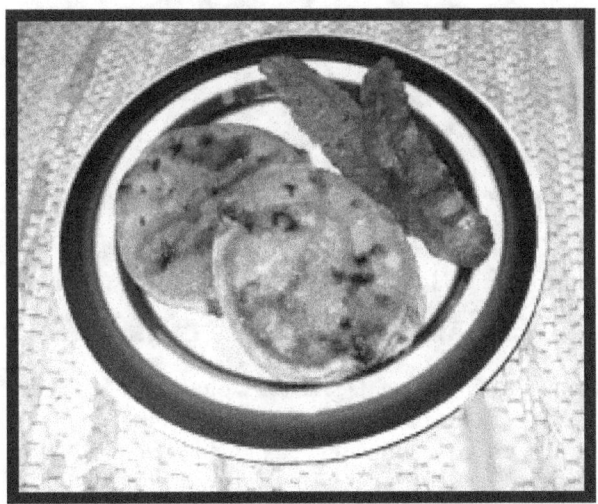

Bacon allowable only on 1500 and 1800 Calorie diets.

<u>Diet Tip of the Day:</u> Most experts associate eating a substantial breakfast with successful weight loss.

Day 11 - Recipe

Artichoke-Bean Salad

    19-ounce can white kidney beans*
    10 artichoke hearts*, quartered
    ⅓ cup chopped oregano
    ⅓ cup chopped parsley
    3 cloves garlic, chopped
    1 lemon, juiced

Combine ingredients in medium-size bowl. Stir in ¼ cup extra-virgin olive oil. Salt and black pepper to taste.
Serves 6. About 190 Calories per serving.

Pictured on the plate below is the artichoke-bean salad as a side dish with two grilled chicken sausage links, tomato salsa and steamed green beans. Incidentally, this artichoke-bean combination over mixed salad greens served with a whole-grain bread makes a delicious, nutritious and reasonable low calorie main course.

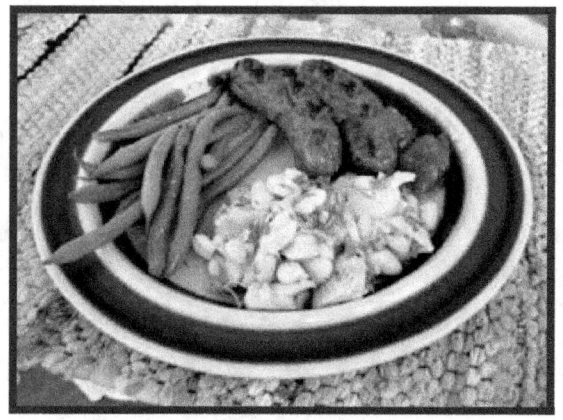

* Canned kidney beans and artichoke hearts should be gluten free but check the ingredients on the container to be sure. Call the manufacturer and ask if the food product could contain trace gluten or could have been cross contaminated in their factory. Do not eat a food if you are not sure it is gluten free. Remember, if in doubt, go without.

Diet Tip of the Day: Before you go to a **party**, have a small meal, such as a hardboiled egg, an apple, and a thirst quencher (like water, tea, seltzer, or diet soda). This will take the edge off your appetite and make it easier to resist the high-calorie goodies.

Day 12 - Recipe

Fish Dinner - Out

No recipe today. No cooking today. Have a fish dinner at a restaurant, but make sure you choose a restaurant where you have a good chance to eat gluten free and achieve your calorie goal. For today, your **goal for dinner is a maximum of 595 Calories**. This includes appetizer, soup, main course and dessert.

Tips for Eating Fish Out: The following is almost an exact repeat of the advice given eating out on previous days. First make sure you choose a restaurant where gluten-free food is available and where you have a good chance to achieve your calorie goal. Before you out go read the menu online and reduce your food choices so you can have more focused questions for the staff. You are more likely to get a safe meal if you call the restaurant before you go to let them know of your gluten-free needs. And call during a slow time so you can have the host's complete attention.

In the restaurant, to ensure you are served a gluten-free meal, it is important to communicate your need to eat 100 percent gluten-free assertively but pleasantly. Try to speak directly to the chef or manager. Otherwise, ask your server what is in the food and how it is prepared. Menu descriptions do not always list every ingredient. Inquire how gluten-free grains such as rice and risottos are cooked. Sometimes they are cooked in broth which may contain gluten. Confirm that separate, clean utensils and equipment will be used to prepare your meal.

Order simple, such as broiled fish with steamed vegetables and brown rice. Tell the waiter you want no sauce, no gravy, nothing added. Then, knowing your calorie objective, and that fish is about 50 Calories per ounce, most steamed vegetable servings average approximately 50 Calories per cup, and rice is about 100 Calories per ½ cup, decide how much to eat – and take the remainder home. And consider bringing your own gluten-free salad dressing to the restaurant. If fresh fruit is not an option, pass on dessert and have the evening snack specified in the *90-Day Gluten-Free Smart Diet* meal plan for that day.

In a restaurant, most nutritionists recommend you eat the low-calorie items on your plate first. Start with the salad, soup and veggies. By the time you get to the chicken and starches you will hopefully be full enough to be content with smaller portions of the higher-calorie choices.

Day 13 - Recipe

<u>Pasta with Marinara Sauce</u>

The spiral pasta profile shown below is called fusilli, a very popular pasta shape because all those ridges hold lots of tomato sauce.

½ small onion, finely chopped
1 teaspoon olive oil
2 garlic cloves, finely chopped
1½ cups chopped plum tomatoes
½ teaspoon chopped fresh oregano
½ pound gluten-free fusilli pasta*
¼ teaspoon salt

Homemade Tomato sauce: Sauté chopped onion in 1 teaspoon olive oil. Add two finely chopped garlic cloves, 1½ cups chopped plum tomatoes and ½ teaspoon chopped fresh oregano. Stir and cook about 5 minutes on a low flame.

Pasta: Bring 2 quarts of lightly salted water to a boil. Add GF pasta and stir occasionally (to keep pasta from sticking to the bottom of the pot). Keep water boiling and cook until pasta are "al dente." (Cooking time is about 9 minutes.) Because the tomato sauce is a bit too thick, add ¼ cup of pasta liquid to the sauce to thin it. Finally drain the pasta, add the marinara sauce and serve hot.

<u>Serves 4.</u> One serving is about 250 Calories.

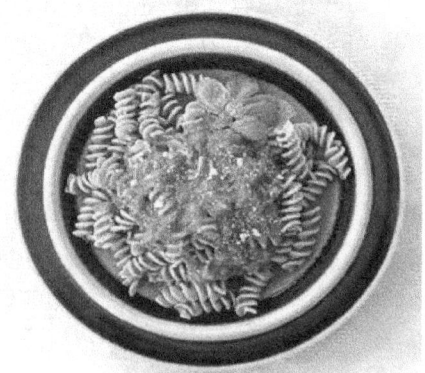

* We used Delallo Whole Grain Rice Fusilli. Chef, Gail Johnson said, "DeLallo pasta is very good with a springy bite and agreeable flavor." See page 223 for additional gluten-free pasta choices.

Day 14 - Recipe

Low-Cal Smoothie

Smoothies are delicious, nutritious and fun to drink! They're great for a fast but nutritious breakfast, a light energy-boosting lunch, a healthy snack, a late afternoon pick me up, and a delicious dessert. Making your own smoothie is a smart way to save money and get healthy at the same time!

- 6 ounces GF plain non-fat yogurt (page 221)
- 1 cup orange juice
- 1 cup strawberries
- ¾ cup blueberries
- 1 banana
- 1 teaspoon sugar
- 1 teaspoon vanilla extract

Place yogurt, strawberries, and blueberries in a blender. Pour in orange juice. Add sugar and vanilla extract to mixture. Blend all ingredients until thick and smooth. Pour smoothie into a glass and enjoy.
Serves 2. About 220 Calories per serving

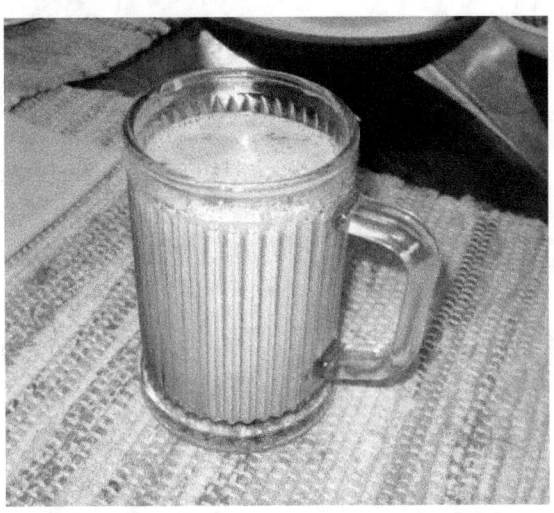

Diet Tip of the Day: Two scientific journals indicate **dark chocolate** - not white chocolate or milk chocolate - is a potent antioxidant and is good for you. But don't overdo it, because you have to offset the extra chocolate calories by eating less of other foods.

Day 15 - Recipe

London Broil

  1 lb boneless flank steak about ¾" thick, fat trimmed
  1 clove garlic
  1 teaspoon dry oregano (See spices page 218)

Rub each side of the flank steak with garlic. Season with oregano, salt and pepper to taste. Prepare a large non-stick skillet over high heat. Steak should sizzle when placed on hot skillet. Sear steak on one side for about 5 minutes; then turn and sear other side for about 4 minutes, or until done to preference. Check the center by making small incision. Carve into ¼-inch slices.

Serves 4. About 320 Calories per serving (for meat only).

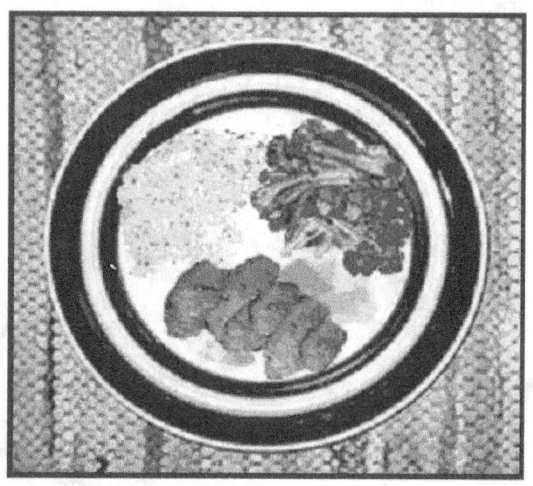

Diet Tip of the Day: Stay Busy. Most people will do anything to avoid work, housework, yard work, exercise, etc. But any kind of work burns a lot more calories than just sitting! Whatever it is you are avoiding – just go do it!

Day 16 - Recipe

Red Snapper with Special Sauce

    4 4-ounce red snapper fillets (salmon fillets also okay)
    ½ cup white wine
    ½ cup GF non-fat yogurt (page 221) mixed with ¼ cup mustard
    ½ pound green beans
    ¾ pint cherry tomatoes (about 20), halved
    4 teaspoons olive oil
    ¾ cup wild rice and brown rice mix.

Brown fillets in non-stick pan. Place fillets skin side down in baking dish coated with non-stick spray. Add white wine and cook in oven preheated to 350 °F for about 15 minutes. Spoon pan juices over fillets. Salt and pepper to taste.

Place green beans in skillet. Add ¼-inch of water and cook over medium heat until water boils off. Add cherry tomatoes and olive oil. Stir well and sauté for a few minutes. (If desired, season with fresh rosemary and oregano.) Salt and pepper to taste.

Prepare rice mix per package directions. Rice is naturally gluten free but check to make sure the rice mix you use is gluten-free.

Plate red snapper fillet and spoon over yogurt-mustard sauce. Add green beans and tomato mix and the wild rice mix. Serve hot.

Serves 4. One plate consisting of one snapper fillet (215 Calories) with green beans and tomato mix (75 Calories) and wild rice (160 Calories) totals 450 Calories.

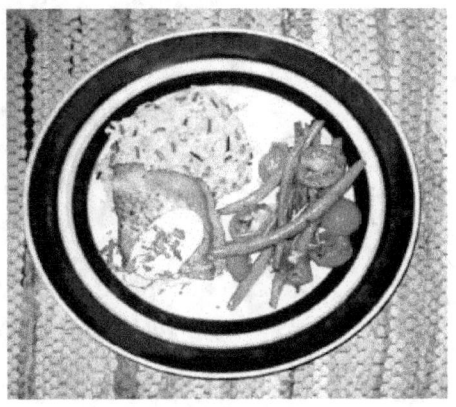

Day 17 - Recipe

Cajun Chicken Salad

This is a perfect after-work, quick, nutritious and delicious dinner.

  4 boneless and skinless chicken breasts - about 5 oz each
  4 teaspoons of bottled Cajun herb-spice (page 223) mix
  8 ounces mixed salad greens
  ¾ pint cherry tomatoes (about 20), halved
  12 pitted black olives
  2 tablespoons bottled lite GF salad dressing

Brush chicken breasts lightly with olive oil. Roll breasts in Cajun herb-spice mix.

Brown breasts on non-stick oven-proof skillet. After breasts are brown, put skillet in 350 ºF oven for approximately 15 minutes, or until done. (When the breasts are done, the meat should be moist and white with no sign of pink.) Cut breasts into ½-inch slices.

Serve hot or keep in an oven or warmer at 200 ºF until ready to plate. Place chicken slices over a bed of mixed salad greens. Add tomatoes, olives and two tablespoons of your favorite lite GF salad dressing. **Serves 4**. 330 Calories per serving

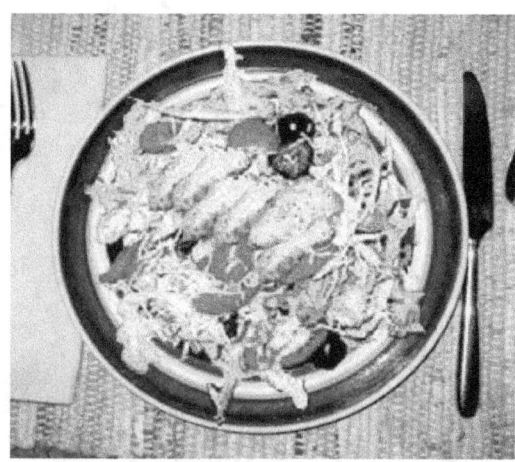

Diet Tip of the Day: Hot or cold cereal topped with fruit, and fat-free milk makes a nutritious, relatively low-calorie meal anytime.

Day 18 - Recipe

Grilled Swordfish

   1 ¼ pounds swordfish
   ¾ pint cherry tomatoes (about 20), halved
   4 medium potatoes
   2 cups fresh spinach
   1 teaspoon rosemary & juice of ¼ lemon
   2 teaspoon extra-virgin olive oil, divided
Steam spinach with garlic and drizzle with about 1 teaspoon extra-virgin olive oil.

Cut potatoes in medium-size pieces and sprinkle with lemon juice, add rosemary, salt and black pepper. Place potatoes on grill for about 10 minutes, turning occasionally. Toss cherry tomatoes in remaining extra-virgin olive oil. Add fresh oregano, salt and black pepper. Place on heavy-duty aluminum foil, seal and grill for about 3 minutes.

GF Lemon-Herb Marinade: 1 lemon - juiced, 1 Tbsp olive oil, 2 garlic cloves minced, 1 tsp fresh thyme chopped, 1 tsp fresh oregano chopped & 1 tsp minced green onion

Immerse swordfish in GF marinade. Grill on hot fire for about 5 minutes on one side and 3 minutes on the other, or until done as desired.
Serves 4. One plate of grilled swordfish (250 Calories) with potatoes (100 Calories), cherry tomatoes (45 Calories) and steamed spinach (50 Calories) totals 445 Calories.

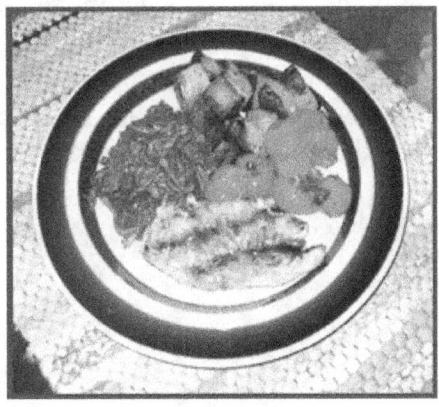

Day 19 - Recipe

Chinese Dinner - Out

No recipe today. No cooking today. Have a Chinese dinner at your favorite restaurant, but make sure you choose a restaurant where you can eat gluten free and have a reasonable chance to achieve your calorie goal. For today, **your goal for dinner is a maximum of 640 Calories**. This includes any appetizer, soup, main course and any dessert.

Tips for Eating Chinese: Try bringing a restaurant card to the Chinese restaurant. The cards are available online and are designed to help explain a gluten-free diet to a waiter who might not speak English.

You can consume a lot of calories in a Chinese restaurant – if you order carelessly. For example a typical portion of General Tso's chicken is loaded with about 1,000 Calories, then add another 200 Calories for a cup of rice.

First rule, order simple. Rice noodles prepared with vegetables or chicken are generally a safe choice. Avoid brown sauce which may have a soy sauce base. Instead, ask for the dish to be prepared with a white sauce using corn starch. Then, knowing your 640 Calorie objective, and that chicken and fish are about 50 Calories per ounce, most steamed vegetable servings average approximately 50 Calories per cup, and rice is about 200 Calories per cup, decide how much of the meal you can eat – and take the remainder home. (Note that you will be eating half a serving of left over Chinese food for lunch tomorrow.) To stay within your maximum allowable calorie total, you should pass on dessert and have the evening snack (if any) specified for that day in the diet.

And although it is customary to share dishes at a Chinese restaurant, do not permit your dinner companions to contaminate your food. Make sure your friends do not use their gluten-contaminated spoons to serve food from your gluten-free dish.

Incidentally, although Chinese is specified, feel free to substitute Thai food, Vietnamese, Indian, Middle Eastern, or any other favorite ethnic food. Just make sure you can eat gluten free and do not exceed the maximum allowable 640 calories for this meal.

Day 20 - Recipe

Quick Pasta alla Puttanesca

This famous pasta dish originated in Naples Italy. Puttanesca means "ladies of the night." Although the exact origin of the name is unclear, one thing is clear: It's delicious! Here is one of many recipe versions.

  ½ pound GF spaghetti (page 222)
  20 black or green pitted olives
  14.5-oz can diced tomatoes
  4 oz GF tomato sauce (page 216)
  2 tablespoon extra-virgin olive oil
  3 cloves of garlic, chopped
  1 tablespoon dried minced onion
  ½ teaspoon crushed red pepper flakes
  1 tablespoon capers drained and rinsed
  ¼ cup currants

Cook spaghetti according to package directions. Drain and return spaghetti to pot; add a teaspoon extra-virgin olive oil and toss to coat.

Heat remaining olive oil in large skillet over medium-high heat. Add red pepper flakes; cook and stir 1 to 2 minutes or until sizzling. Add onion and garlic; cook and stir 1 minute. Add canned tomatoes with juice, tomato sauce, olives, currants and capers. Cook over medium-high heat, stirring frequently, until sauce is heated through.
Serves 4. About 345 Calories per serving

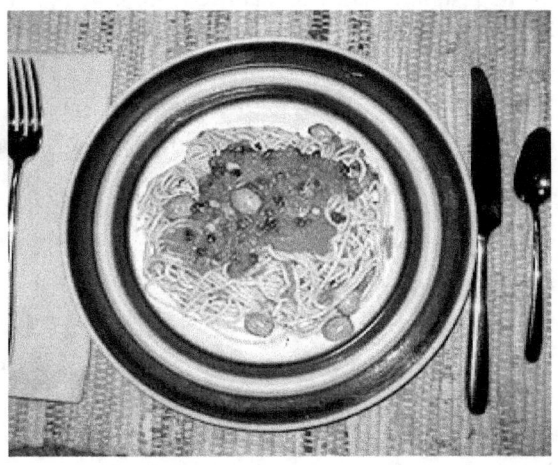

Day 21 - Recipe

Frozen Dinner

No recipe today. No cooking today. It's your day off! At this writing, Amy's and Artisan Bistro offer quite a few gluten-free frozen entrees. Smart Ones only makes two gluten-free entrees. Glutino also makes two gluten-free frozen entrees, but each contain 400 Calories, and are not included in the following list.

- Amy's Quinoa, Black Beans, Butternut Squash & Chard (**240 Cal**)
- Amy's Black Bean & Cheese Enchilada (**240 Cal**)
- Amy's Mushroom Risotto Bowl (**240 Cal**)
- Amy's Sweet & Sour Asian Noodle Bowl (**250 Cal**)
- Amy's Vegetable Parmesan Bowl (**260 Cal**)
- Amy's Brown Rice & Veggies Bowl – Light in Sodium (**260 Cal**)
- Amy's Brown Rice, Black-eyed Peas & Veggies Bowl (**290 Cal**)
- Amy's Teriyaki Bowl (**290 Cal**)
- Amy's Asian Noodle Stir Fry (**300 Cal**)
- Amy's Vegetable Lasagna (**300 Cal**)
- Amy's Thai Stir-Fry (**310 Cal**)
- Amy's Tofu Scramble (**320 Cal**)

- Artisan Bistro Wild Alaskan Salmon (**200 Cal**)
- Artisan Bistro Chicken Parmesan Bake (**200 Cal**)
- Artisan Bistro Turkey Cheddar Bake (**240 Cal**)
- Artisan Bistro Wild Alaskan Salmon Bake (**240 Cal**)
- Artisan Bistro Thai Style Yellow Curry with Chicken (**240 Cal**)
- Artisan Bistro Cheddar Beef Bake (**250 Cal**)
- Artisan Bistro Sesame Ginger with Salmon (**270 Cal**)
- Artisan Bistro Coconut Lemongrass with Chicken (**270 Cal**)
- Artisan Bistro Spiced Chicken Morocco (**270 Cal**)
- Artisan Bistro Albacore Tuna Bake (**280 Cal**)
- Artisan Bistro Thai Style Red Curry with Beef (**280 Cal**)
- Artisan Bistro Chicken Citron (**280 Cal**)
- Artisan Bistro Wild Alaskan Salmon with Pesto (**310 Cal**)
- Artisan Bistro Savory Turkey (**330 Cal**)
- Artisan Bistro Southwest Style Beef (**330 Cal**)
- Artisan Bistro Ginger Chicken (**350 Cal**)
- Artisan Bistro Beef with Mushroom Sauce (**350 Cal**)
- Artisan Bistro Wild Alaskan Salmon Cake (**370 Cal**)

- Smart Ones Lemon Herb Chicken Piccata (**250 Cal**)
- Smart Ones Santa Fe Style Rice & Beans (**290 Cal**)

That's it. There are just not many low-calorie frozen GF entrees currently in stores. But more food manufacturers are getting on the GF band wagon, so check your local supermarket for the latest gluten-free frozen entrees. Also note that **340 Calories are allocated for this meal**. But almost all of the above have less than 340 Calories. Use the excess calories anyway you wish. Splurge on extra dessert or save the calories for another day! And please read the important **Frozen-Food Safety Warning** in **Appendix D** (page 226).

<u>**Diet Tip of the Day:**</u> **Understanding nutrition** is not only vital for good health but also will help you control your weight over the long term. For example, did you know that foods that are labeled an "excellent source" of a particular nutrient provide 20% or more of the Recommended Daily Value. Whereas, foods that are a "good source" of a nutrient provide between 10 and 20% of the Recommended Daily Value.

Day 22 - Recipe

<u>Shrimp & Spinach Salad</u>

  2 pounds shrimp in shell
  ½ pound small green beans, trimmed
  ½ pound baby spinach leaves
  2 tablespoon lemon juice
  ¼ cup extra-virgin olive oil
  2 teaspoon minced fresh dill
  1 tablespoon minced green onion

To make vinaigrette, combine lemon juice, olive oil, dill, salt and black pepper to taste and whisk until blended. Stir in minced onion and set aside. Steam green beans and set aside.

Peel, de-vein and butterfly shrimp. Place shrimp in a bowl and add water to cover. Add 1 teaspoon of salt, and let stand for 10 minutes. Drain, rinse, drain again, and dry. Arrange shrimp in broiling pan without a rack. Brush shrimp with a little of the vinaigrette and place under preheated broiler, about 3 inches from heat. Broil about 3 to 4 minutes, turning shrimp once, or until both sides turn pink.

Remove shrimp from broiler and add remaining vinaigrette and green beans to the broiling pan. Stir to coat shrimp and beans with vinaigrette. Pour warm vinaigrette over spinach and toss quickly. Plate the spinach and arrange shrimp and green beans on top.
Serves 4. 310 Calories per serving.

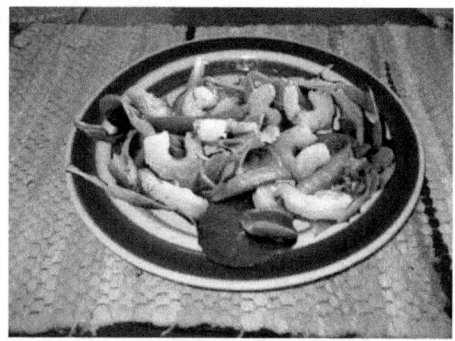

Diet Tip of the Day: After company leaves, have them take some of the leftover food (particularly the dessert) with them – or take the leftovers to work the next day.

Day 23 - Recipe

<u>Beans & Greens Salad</u>

⅓ cup chopped oregano
⅓ cup chopped parsley
3 cloves garlic, chopped
1 lemon, juiced

Prepare dressing by combining above ingredients and stirring in ¼ cup extra-virgin olive oil. Salt and black pepper to taste.

½ pound mesclun mix
¼ pound green beans
19-oz can garbanzo beans (chickpeas)*

Arrange mesclun mix, garbanzo beans and green beans on large platter. Drizzle dressing over beans and greens.

<u>Serves 4</u>. Approximately 260 Calories per serving.

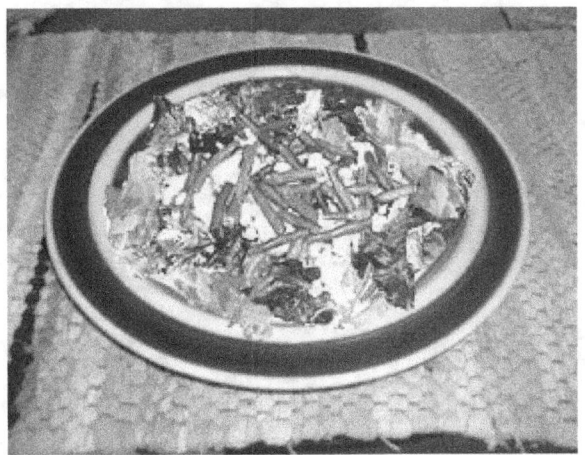

* Canned garbanzo beans should be gluten free but check the ingredients on the container to be sure. Call the manufacturer and ask if the food product could contain trace gluten or could have been cross contaminated in their factory. Do not eat a food if you are not sure it is gluten free. Remember, if in doubt, go without.

<u>Diet Tip of the Day:</u> Beans are a wonderful food but **beans are an incomplete protein**. If however beans are eaten with a whole-grain bread, the combination forms a complete protein – just as complete and nutritious as meat, poultry, or fish.

Day 24- Recipe

Four-Bean Plus Salad (This is a side dish)

Note that the total caloric value of the salad will change very little, if the proportions of the bean varieties and corn are varied – according to taste. But make sure all the canned foods are gluten free.

- ½ cup canned red kidney beans*, drained and rinsed
- ½ cup canned black beans*, drained and rinsed
- ½ cup canned chick peas*, drained and rinsed
- ½ cup canned cannelloni beans*, drained and rinsed
- ½ cup canned corn, drained
- 1 small red pepper, chopped
- 1 small green pepper, chopped
- 2 tablespoons extra-virgin olive oil
- 2 tablespoons lemon juice

In a large bowl mix red kidney beans, black beans, chick peas, cannelloni beans, corn and chopped red and green peppers. Stir in olive oil and lemon juice and plate.

Serves about 6. One serving is ½ cup – with about 135 Calories per serving

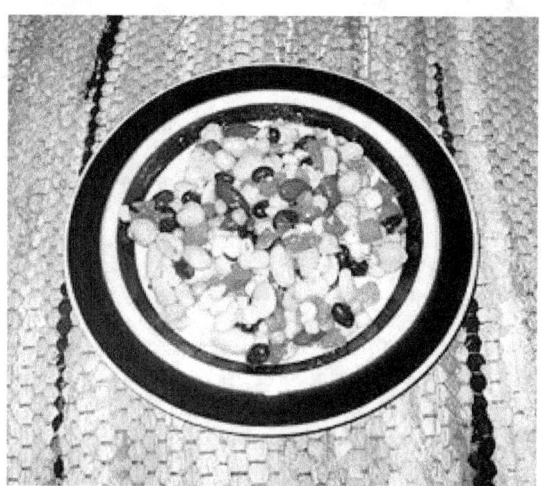

* Canned red kidney beans, black beans, chick peas and cannelloni beans should be gluten free but check the ingredients on the container to be sure. Call the manufacturer and ask if the food product could contain trace gluten or could have been cross contaminated in their factory. Do not eat a food if you are not sure it is gluten free. Remember, if in doubt, go without.

Day 25 - Recipe

<u>Pan-Broiled Hanger Steak</u>

1¼ pounds hanger steak, well trimmed of fat
¼ cup lime juice
8 small new potatoes, peeled and halved
½ pint cherry tomatoes (about 15), halved

Season both sides of steak with salt and pepper and place in sealable plastic bag with lime juice. Refrigerate for about one hour.

Boil potatoes about 10 minutes. Rinse in cold water. Sauté potatoes in small amount of vegetable oil over medium-high heat until brown.

Sauté cherry tomatoes in small amount of olive oil over medium-high heat until skin begins to crack. Season with chopped fresh basil.

Heat a skillet over medium-high heat. Sear hanger steak on one side for about 5 minutes. Turn over and sear other side approximately 5 minutes (for medium done). Pour off any fat that may have accumulated. Cut into ½-inch slices.

<u>Serves 4.</u> About 320 Calories per serving (for the hanger steak only)

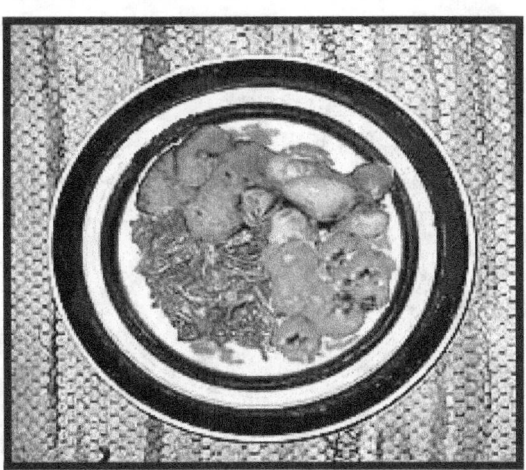

<u>Diet Tip of the Day:</u> If you go to a **party**, don't stand near the food! Be aware of the temptation. Make the effort, and you'll find you eat less.

Day 26 - Recipe

Tina's Grilled Scallops &Polenta

1 pound sea scallops
¾ cup GF polenta (page 216)
¾ cup skim milk
1 medium portobello mushroom
½ pound green beans
¼ cup chopped red onion
16 asparagus spear
1 teaspoon extra-virgin olive oil

Bring 1½ cups of water and skim milk to rapid boil. Add salt to taste and slowly add GF polenta while stirring. Reduce heat. Continue stirring until desired consistency is reached. Pour polenta into lightly greased pan. After polenta has cooled cover and refrigerate. Cut chilled polenta into 4 pieces. Grill on medium-hot fire – about two minutes on each side.

Brush portobello mushroom and asparagus spear with olive oil and place on grill for about 3 minutes on each side.

Grill scallops on medium-hot fire. Turn after two minutes or when first side turns opaque. Grill until second side turns opaque – about another 2 minutes. Don't overcook but test a scallop by cutting to make sure it's cooked through. Salt and pepper to taste.

Serves 4. The food on the plate pictured below totals about 380 Calories.

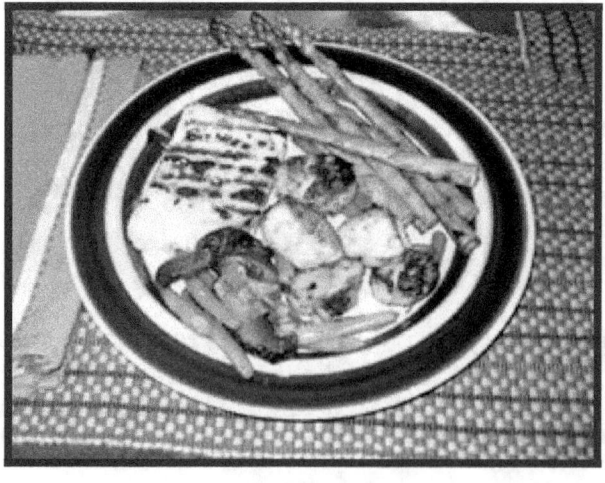

Day 27 - Recipe

Fettuccine in Summer Sauce

This sauce is often served in the summer because it's lighter than what is usually dished up with pasta. But despite its name the sauce is wonderful year round.

½ lb GF fettuccine pasta*
8 oz fresh asparagus, trimmed & cut in 2-inch pieces
¾ pint cherry tomatoes (about 20), halved
2 Tbsp plus 1 tsp extra-virgin olive oil, divided
2 cloves of garlic, chopped
½ small onion, diced

Cook GF fettuccine according to package directions. Drain and return pasta to pot; add a teaspoon of the olive oil and toss to coat. Meanwhile steam asparagus and drain.

In large skillet over medium-high heat, sauté cherry tomatoes in remaining 2 tablespoons of olive oil until skin begins to crack. Add onion and cook until translucent. Stir in garlic. Thin sauce with pasta liquid to desired consistency. Toss cooked pasta and asparagus into sauce and serve.

Serves 4. About 290 Calories per serving

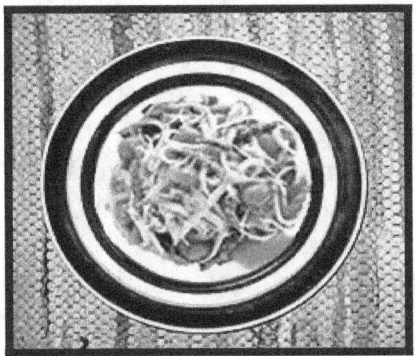

* If you cannot find gluten-free fettuccine, substitute any other shape of GF pasta.

Diet Tip of the Day: A major weight-loss fallacy is that you can **get rid of abdominal fat** by working your abdominal muscles. This is based on the incorrect belief that fat is eliminated from a particular part of your body if you engage the muscles underneath that layer of fat. No such luck.

Day 28 - Recipe

Frozen Dinner

No recipe today. No cooking today. It's your day off! At this writing, Amy's and Artisan Bistro offer quite a few gluten-free frozen entrees. Smart Ones only makes two gluten-free entrees.

- Amy's Quinoa, Black Beans, Butternut Squash & Chard (**240 Cal**)
- Amy's Black Bean & Cheese Enchilada (**240 Cal**)
- Amy's Mushroom Risotto Bowl (**240 Cal**)
- Amy's Sweet & Sour Asian Noodle Bowl (**250 Cal**)
- Amy's Vegetable Parmesan Bowl (**260 Cal**)
- Amy's Brown Rice & Veggies Bowl – Light in Sodium (**260 Cal**)
- Amy's Brown Rice, Black-eyed Peas & Veggies Bowl (**290 Cal**)
- Amy's Teriyaki Bowl (**290 Cal**)
- Amy's Asian Noodle Stir Fry (**300 Cal**)
- Amy's Vegetable Lasagna (**300 Cal**)
- Amy's Thai Stir-Fry (**310 Cal**)
- Amy's Tofu Scramble (**320 Cal**)

- Artisan Bistro Wild Alaskan Salmon (**200 Cal**)
- Artisan Bistro Chicken Parmesan Bake (**200 Cal**)
- Artisan Bistro Turkey Cheddar Bake (**240 Cal**)
- Artisan Bistro Wild Alaskan Salmon Bake (**240 Cal**)
- Artisan Bistro Thai Style Yellow Curry with Chicken (**240 Cal**)
- Artisan Bistro Cheddar Beef Bake (**250 Cal**)
- Artisan Bistro Sesame Ginger with Salmon (**270 Cal**)
- Artisan Bistro Coconut Lemongrass with Chicken (**270 Cal**)
- Artisan Bistro Spiced Chicken Morocco (**270 Cal**)
- Artisan Bistro Albacore Tuna Bake (**280 Cal**)
- Artisan Bistro Thai Style Red Curry with Beef (**280 Cal**)
- Artisan Bistro Chicken Citron (**280 Cal**)
- Artisan Bistro Wild Alaskan Salmon with Pesto (**310 Cal**)
- Artisan Bistro Savory Turkey (**330 Cal**)
- Artisan Bistro Southwest Style Beef (**330 Cal**)
- Artisan Bistro Ginger Chicken (**350 Cal**)
- Artisan Bistro Beef with Mushroom Sauce (**350 Cal**)
- Artisan Bistro Wild Alaskan Salmon Cake (**370 Cal**)

- Smart Ones Lemon Herb Chicken Piccata (**250 Cal**)

- Smart Ones Santa Fe Style Rice & Beans (**290 Cal**)

Also note that **340 Calories are allocated for this meal**. But almost all of the above have less than 340 Calories. Use the excess calories anyway you wish. Splurge on extra dessert or save the calories for another day!

And please read the important **Frozen-Food Safety Warning** in **Appendix D** (page 226).

Day 29 - Recipe

<u>Barbequed Shrimp & Corn</u>

    1 ½ pounds large shrimp, peeled and de-veined
    3 Tbsp of bottled GF barbeque sauce (page 217)
    4 medium ears of corn

Pour barbeque sauce into shallow bowl. Toss shrimp in barbeque sauce to coat. Place shrimp on medium-hot grill. Turn shrimp after about two minutes or when shrimp turn pink. Grill until second side turns pink – approximately another 2 minutes. Don't overcook but test a shrimp by cutting to make sure it is cooked through. Salt and pepper to taste. Serve hot or at room temperature.
<u>Serves 4</u>. About 160 Calories per serving (shrimp only).

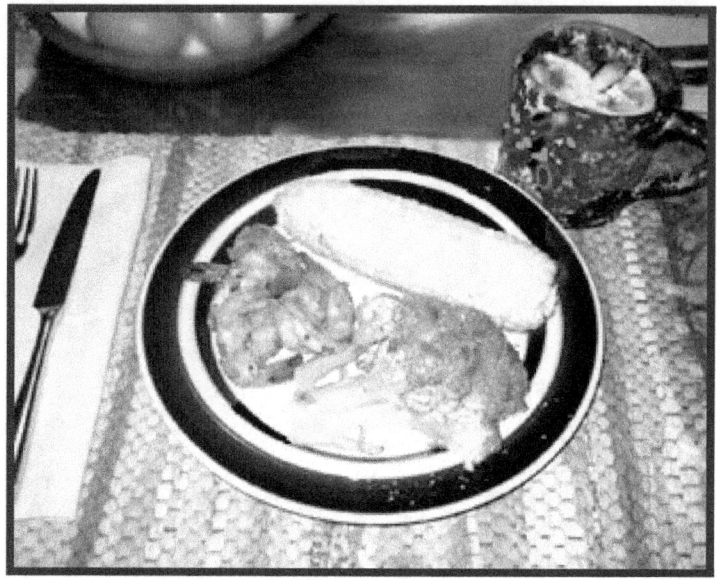

<u>Diet Tip of the Day:</u> A very **important weight-profile parameter** is your waist-to-hip ratio. Health risks for heart attack and stroke increase considerably for men with a ratio above 1.0 and for women with a ratio above 0.8. To calculate your ratio, measure your waist size (at its narrowest circumference) and divide it by your hip size (at the widest section).

Day 30 - Recipe

<u>Cheeseburger Heaven</u>

There's really not much to grilling hamburgers. The ideal meat for a juicy burger is ground chuck with about 20% fat, but we are talking diet here. So we opt for leaner, much leaner meat.

    1¼ pounds ground sirloin (95% lean)
    4 thin slices light GF cheese (page 221)

Mix ground beef in large bowl. Salt and pepper to taste. Divide into 4 equal portions and form burgers about 1-inch thick.

Cook burgers over a hot fire on charcoal or gas-fired grill. For medium, cook about 4 minutes on each side. Top with slice of light GF cheese. Add lettuce and tomato. Season to taste.

<u>Serves 4</u>. About 320 Calories per serving (cheeseburger only).

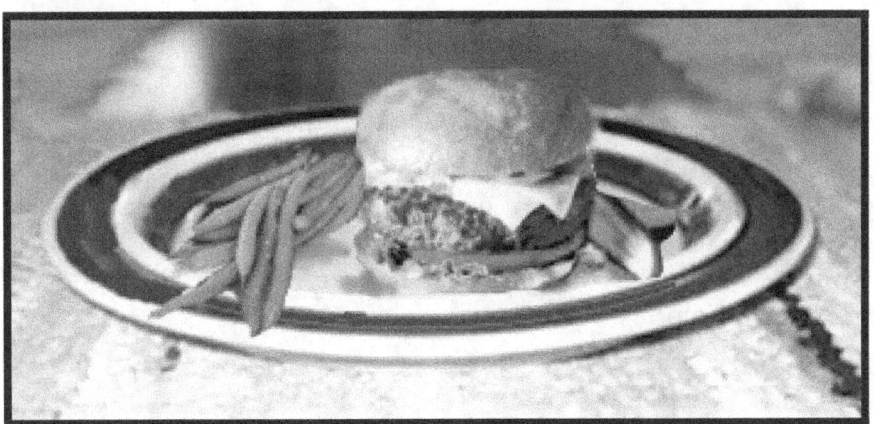

<u>Diet Tip of the Day:</u> **Plan to be on a diet the rest of your life**. Not necessarily a weight reducing diet. At some point you'll want to just maintain your weight. But you will still need to continue to make good healthy food choices – and not slip back to your old eating habits.

Day 31 - Recipe

<u>Tina's Baked Sea Bass</u>

    4 4-ounce Chilean sea bass fillets
    ½ pound green beans
    ¾ pint cherry tomatoes (about 20)
    ¾ cup brown rice (prepare per package directions)

<u>Sea Bass:</u> Dust filets with GF all purpose flour (page 215). Dip in egg wash and then GF Panko bread crumbs (page 216). Place fillets in baking dish coated with non-stick spray. Bake about 15 minutes in oven preheated to 350 °F.

<u>Green Beans & Tomato:</u> Place green beans in skillet. Add ¼-inch of water and cook over medium heat until water boils off. Add cherry tomatoes and olive oil. Stir well and sauté for a few minutes. Season with fresh rosemary and oregano.

<u>Brown Rice-Pesto mix:</u> Prepare brown rice per package directions. Add 4 teaspoons packaged "green" pesto*. Mix thoroughly.

<u>Red Pepper Sauce:</u> Blend one roasted red pepper (skinned), ½ cup GF non-fat plain yogurt, 1 tsp lemon juice, 1 Tbsp olive oil, 1 Tbsp chili sauce, and a dash of Worcestershire sauce (page 218).

<u>Serves 4</u>. One plate consisting of one sea bass fillet with spooned over red pepper sauce (150 Calories), green beans & tomato mix (75 Calories), brown rice-pesto mix (120 Calories) and half ear of corn (50 Calories) – totals about 395 Calories.

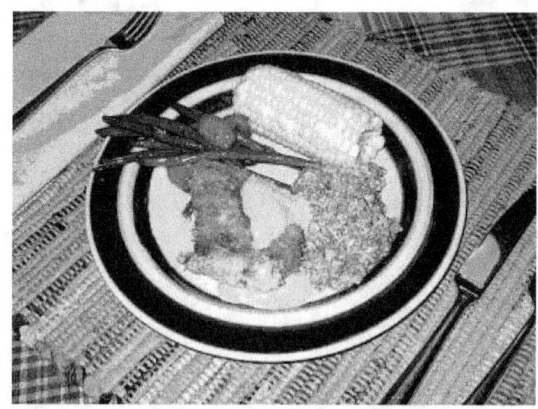

* Naturally gluten-free, pesto is a traditional northern Italian sauce. Pesto, meaning "pounded" in Italian and traditionally is made with fresh basil, Parmesan cheese, olive oil, pine nuts and garlic.

Day 32 - Recipe

Turkey Tenders & Vegetables

 2 turkey breast tenderloins (about 1½ lb)
 1 medium eggplant (about ¾ lb)
 ¾ pound yellow (summer) squash
 2 medium plum tomatoes, quartered

Marinade: Whisk in a bowl 2 tsp lemon zest, ¼ cup lemon juice, 2 Tbsp olive oil, 1 Tbsp chopped garlic, 1 Tbsp chopped rosemary, ¼ tsp salt and a pinch of black pepper. Put marinade and turkey breasts in large re-sealable plastic bag. Refrigerate about 45 minutes

Slice eggplant and squash lengthwise about ½-inch thick. Place with tomatoes on a baking sheet coated with a nonstick spray.

Grill turkey breasts approximately 7 to 9 minutes per side, or until an instant-read thermometer inserted from the side to middle registers 160°F. Slice turkey and set aside.

Grill eggplant and zucchini about 4 minutes per side, or until just tender. Grill tomatoes about 2 minutes per side, or until charred but not soft. Cut vegetables bite-size and toss with remaining marinade. Serve with sliced turkey.

Serves 4. About 350 Calories per serving (includes turkey and veggies)

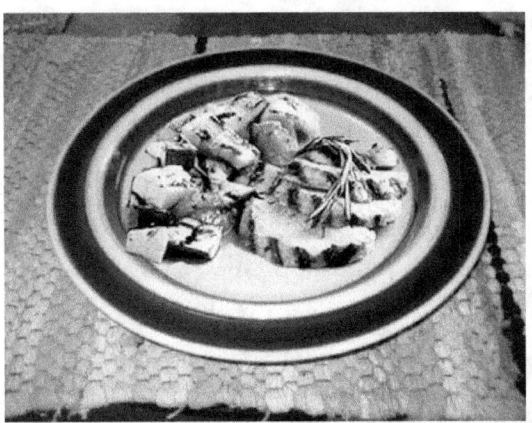

Diet Tip of the Day: It's a lot easier to eat 1000 Calories than it is to burn 1000 Calories exercising. So a stroll after dinner is not going to offset the calories you ingested eating a Big Mac plus fries.

Day 33 - Recipe

Frozen Dinner

No recipe today. No cooking today. It's your day off! At this writing, Amy's and Artisan Bistro offer quite a few gluten-free frozen entrees. Smart Ones only makes two gluten-free entrees. Glutino also makes two gluten-free frozen entrees, but each contain 400 Calories, and are not included in the following list.

- Amy's Quinoa, Black Beans, Butternut Squash & Chard (**240 Cal**)
- Amy's Black Bean & Cheese Enchilada (**240 Cal**)
- Amy's Mushroom Risotto Bowl (**240 Cal**)
- Amy's Sweet & Sour Asian Noodle Bowl (**250 Cal**)
- Amy's Vegetable Parmesan Bowl (**260 Cal**)
- Amy's Brown Rice & Veggies Bowl – Light in Sodium (**260 Cal**)
- Amy's Brown Rice, Black-eyed Peas & Veggies Bowl (**290 Cal**)
- Amy's Teriyaki Bowl (**290 Cal**)
- Amy's Asian Noodle Stir Fry (**300 Cal**)
- Amy's Vegetable Lasagna (**300 Cal**)
- Amy's Thai Stir-Fry (**310 Cal**)
- Amy's Tofu Scramble (**320 Cal**)

- Artisan Bistro Wild Alaskan Salmon (**200 Cal**)
- Artisan Bistro Chicken Parmesan Bake (**200 Cal**)
- Artisan Bistro Turkey Cheddar Bake (**240 Cal**)
- Artisan Bistro Wild Alaskan Salmon Bake (**240 Cal**)
- Artisan Bistro Thai Style Yellow Curry with Chicken (**240 Cal**)
- Artisan Bistro Cheddar Beef Bake (**250 Cal**)
- Artisan Bistro Sesame Ginger with Salmon (**270 Cal**)
- Artisan Bistro Coconut Lemongrass with Chicken (**270 Cal**)
- Artisan Bistro Spiced Chicken Morocco (**270 Cal**)
- Artisan Bistro Albacore Tuna Bake (**280 Cal**)
- Artisan Bistro Thai Style Red Curry with Beef (**280 Cal**)
- Artisan Bistro Chicken Citron (**280 Cal**)
- Artisan Bistro Wild Alaskan Salmon with Pesto (**310 Cal**)
- Artisan Bistro Savory Turkey (**330 Cal**)
- Artisan Bistro Southwest Style Beef (**330 Cal**)
- Artisan Bistro Ginger Chicken (**350 Cal**)
- Artisan Bistro Beef with Mushroom Sauce (**350 Cal**)
- Artisan Bistro Wild Alaskan Salmon Cake (**370 Cal**)

- Smart Ones Lemon Herb Chicken Piccata (**250 Cal**)
- Smart Ones Santa Fe Style Rice & Beans (**290 Cal**)

Also note that **340 Calories are allocated for this meal**. But almost all of the above have less than 340 Calories. Use the excess calories anyway you wish. Splurge on extra dessert or save the calories for another day!

And please read the important **Frozen-Food Safety Warning** in **Appendix D** (page 226).

<u>**Diet Tip of the Day:**</u> It's amazing how many people tend to confuse thirst with hunger. This often results in overeating when actually drinking water might be the solution. So, the next time you have a seemingly uncontrollable food craving, try drinking a glass of water instead.

Pasta Rapini

    2 cloves garlic - coarsely chopped
    1½ cups of crushed tomatoes (San Marzano preferred)
    2 cups Rapini (broccoli rabe)
    1 tablespoon crushed red pepper flakes (optional)
    ½ pound medium-sized GF spaghetti

Tomato Sauce: In large pan, sauté two tablespoons olive oil over medium-high heat. Add the garlic and sauté until translucent (but not browned). Add crushed San Marzano tomatoes (use plum tomatoes if San Marzano are not available) and bring to a boil. Reduce heat to low and simmer for about 30 minutes or until cooked. Season with salt and pepper. Set aside.

Rapini: Discard the tough stems and slice into 2-inch pieces. Bring a pot of water to a boil. Add Rapini (a variety of broccoli rabe) and 1 tablespoon salt. Blanch Rapini about 5 minutes or until slightly cooked but still crunchy at stems. Drain, set aside and cover.

Cook pasta according to package instructions until al dente. Three minutes before pasta is ready, add the Rapini to the sauté pan (containing the tomato sauce). Heat mixture over medium heat. Drain pasta and add it to the pan with the Rapini and tomatoes. Add hot pepper flakes (optional) and toss for 1 to 2 minutes over high heat. Drizzle lightly with extra virgin olive oil and plate. Delicious!
Serves 4. About 290 Calories per serving

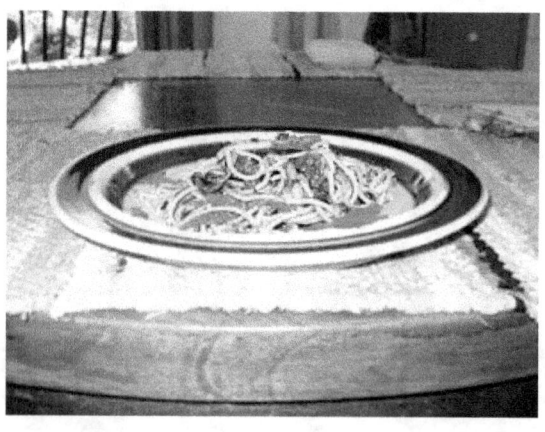

Day 35 - Recipe

<u>Chicken Dinner - Out</u>

No recipe today. No cooking today. Today you eat at a restaurant. But when you are on a gluten-free reducing diet, eating in a restaurant can be a double challenge. First, most restaurant portions are huge, easily totaling more than 1,000 Calories, and then many restaurants do not offer gluten-free menu selections. On the *90-Day Gluten-Free Smart Diet*, a dinner type (i.e., fish, chicken, etc) and a calorie target are specified. For example Day 35 of the 1,200 Calorie diet calls for a chicken dinner and allows you 530 Calories for appetizer, soup, main course and dessert. Follow these tips to make sure your dinning experience is low calorie, gluten-free and pleasant.

Make sure you choose a restaurant where gluten-free food is available and where you have a fighting chance to achieve your calorie goal. Before you out go read the menu online and reduce your food choices so you can have more focused questions for the staff. You are more likely to get a safe meal if you call the restaurant before you go to let them know of your gluten-free needs. And call during a slow time so you can have the host's complete attention.

In the restaurant, to ensure you are served a gluten-free meal, it is important to communicate your need to eat 100 percent gluten-free assertively but amiably. Try to speak directly to the chef or manager. Otherwise, ask your server what is in the food and how it is prepared. Menu descriptions do not always list every ingredient. Inquire how gluten-free grains such as rice and risottos are cooked. Sometimes they are cooked in broth which may contain gluten. Confirm that separate, clean utensils and equipment will be used to prepare your meal.

Order something simple, such as skinless white meat broiled chicken breast with steamed vegetables and brown rice. Tell the waiter you want no sauce, no gravy, nothing added. Then, knowing your calorie objective, and that most fish and chicken are about 50 Calories per ounce, most steamed vegetable servings average approximately 50 Calories per cup, and rice is about 100 Calories per ½ cup, decide how much to eat – and take the remainder home. And consider bringing your own gluten-free salad dressing to the restaurant.   If fresh fruit is not an option, pass on dessert and have the evening snack specified in the *90-Day Gluten-Free Smart Diet* meal plan for that day.

In a restaurant, most nutritionists recommend you eat the low calorie items on your plate first. Start with the salad, soup and veggies. By the time you get to the chicken and starches you will hopefully be full enough to be content with smaller portions of the higher-calorie choices. (Incidentally, feel free to substitute skinless white meat turkey for chicken.)

Diet Tip of the Day: To determine your frame size, circle your wrist with your thumb and third finger. If the tips of your fingers overlap, you have a small frame. If they just touch you are medium, and if they don't touch you have a large frame.

Day 36 - Recipe

Grilled Tilapia

Tilapia is a mild white fish that inhabits fresh water. This fish has very low levels of mercury because it's fast-growing, short-lived, and is eats mostly vegetarian. According to the Monterey Bay Aquarium, choose tilapia farmed in the U.S., in environmentally friendly systems. Avoid farmed tilapia from China and Taiwan, where pollution and weak management are a problem.

4 Tilapia filets (about 6 ounces each)

Marinade: ¾ cup olive oil, ½ lemon, juiced, 1 tablespoons oregano, ½ teaspoon black pepper, ¼ cup red wine vinegar, ½ cup finely chopped parsley and 2 cloves garlic, minced. Combine all marinade ingredients in a large re-sealable plastic bag and shake well.

Place fish filets in the marinade for 30 minutes. Remove fillets from marinade and cook on hot grill for approximately 2 to 3 minutes per side.

Serves 4. About 300 Calories per serving (fish only)

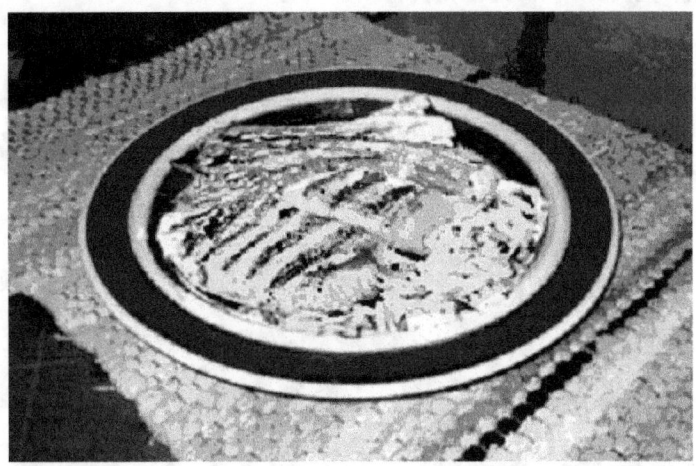

Photo shows two fish filets. Actual serving size is one filet.

Diet Tip of the Day: One serving of asparagus can provide you with 66% of your daily folate needs. Folate is a B-vitamin which is involved with cellular division, and therefore aids the development of a baby's nervous system.

Day 37 - Recipe

Lo-Cal Beef Stew

- ½ lb beef stew meat, fat trimmed & cut in 1" cubes
- 2 celery stalks diced
- 1 medium onion diced
- 3 large carrots cut into large chunks
- 3 large boiling potatoes, peeled & cut in chunks
- ½ up green beans
- 8 ounces GF beef stock (page 223)
- 2 tablespoons of flour, and 1 tablespoon of olive oil
- ½ teaspoon dried herbs, and 1 bay leaf

Season meat with ½ teaspoon dried herbs, salt and pepper. In a Dutch oven, add olive oil and heat until warm. Add meat, diced onion and celery and cook over medium heat about 5 minutes. Add enough GF beef stock to cover meat. Bring to a boil. Reduce heat, add bay leaf, cover and simmer over low heat until meat is fork tender (about 1½ hours). Add potatoes and carrots. Cover and cook until vegetables are tender (about 30 min). Add green beans and cook an additional 10 min. Skim off any fat from the surface.

In a small bowl, add small amount of water to 2 tablespoons of GF all purpose flour (page 215) – and stir. Pour the flour-water mixture into the stew and stir until a thick gravy forms. Taste and adjust seasoning. Spoon approximately ¼ of the stew into each bowl.
Serves 4. About 365 Calories per serving

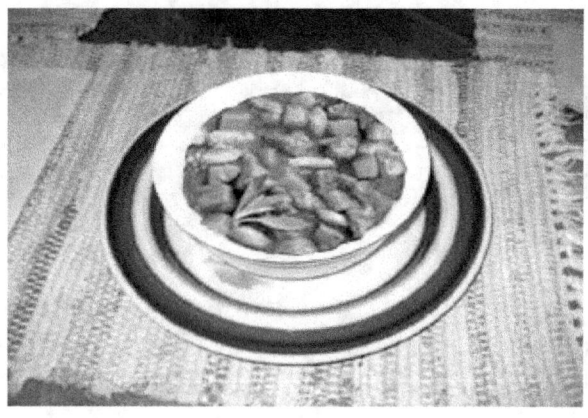

Day 38 - Recipe

<u>Pan-Broiled Lamb Chop</u>

Pan broiling is a quick, easy and a relatively low-calorie technique that can be used to cook many meats.

Start with a rib lamb chop about ¾-inch thick that weighs roughly 6 ounces. Next, it is very important to carefully trim all the visible fat. (After removing the fat and accounting for the bone, about 4 ounces of lean meat should remain.)

Season the chop with salt and ground black pepper. Heat a well-seasoned cast iron or nonstick skillet over high heat. Add the chop (or chops) and cook approximately 4 minutes on each side. (Check center of chop with a small incision to determine when the meat is done.) Plate and serve immediately.

<u>Serves 1</u>: About 320 Calories per chop

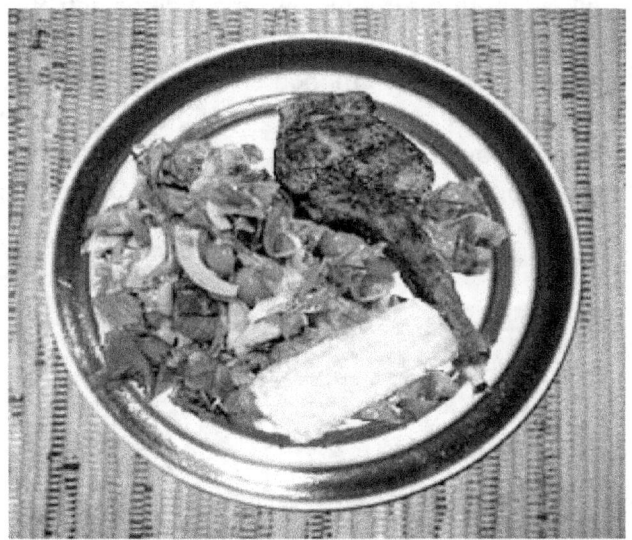

Note corn-on-the-cob is only for the 1800-Calorie diet.

<u>Diet Tip of the Day:</u> According to a study published in the Journal of Food Chemistry, broccoli, spinach, kale, Brussels sprouts and other dark green vegetables have the highest cancer-fighting potential found in produce.

Day 39 - Recipe

Chicken with Veggies

  4 boneless, skinless chicken breast halves (about 5 oz each)
 12 broccoli florets
  1 bunch of asparagus
  2 ripe medium-size tomatoes
  2 tablespoons GF lite salad dressing

Place evenly cut broccoli and asparagus spear in a microwave-safe pan, add a little water to bottom of the pan and top with microwave-safe plastic wrap. (Be sure to pull back one corner of the plastic topper so some steam can escape.) Check veggies periodically and take them out of the microwave when they reach desired softness.

Season chicken breasts evenly with salt and pepper. Heat a large nonstick skillet over medium-high heat. Coat pan with cooking spray. Cook chicken about 4 minutes on each side or until no pink remains.

For each serving, plate one chicken breast and a portion of the steamed broccoli and asparagus. Add one-half of a tomato cut into pieces. Drizzle about 2 tablespoons of GF lite salad dressing (page 222) that contains no more than 25 Calories per tablespoon.
Serves 4: One serving of chicken breast halve, veggies & dressing is about 365 Calories.

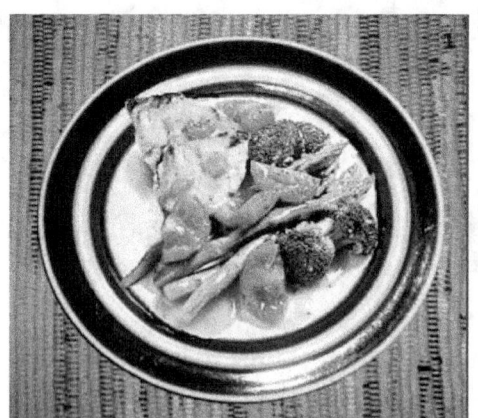

Shown drizzled with Light Thousand Island dressing.

Diet Tip of the Day: Steaming in a microwave oven is one of the best ways to cook veggies so they retain nutrients. Another advantage is the cooking adds no fat or sodium.

Day 40 - Recipe

Fish Dinner - Out

No recipe today. No cooking today. Have a fish dinner at a restaurant, but make sure you choose a restaurant where you have a good chance to eat gluten free and achieve your calorie goal. For today, your **goal for dinner is a maximum of 595 Calories**. This includes appetizer, soup, main course and dessert.

Tips for Eating Fish Out: The following is almost an exact repeat of the advice given eating out on previous days. First make sure you choose a restaurant where gluten-free food is available and where you have a good chance to achieve your calorie goal. Before you out go read the menu online and reduce your food choices so you can have more focused questions for the staff. You are more likely to get a safe meal if you call the restaurant before you go to let them know of your gluten-free needs. And call during a slow time so you can have the host's complete attention.

In the restaurant, to ensure you are served a gluten-free meal, it is important to communicate your need to eat 100 percent gluten-free assertively but pleasantly. Try to speak directly to the chef or manager. Otherwise, ask your server what is in the food and how it is prepared. Menu descriptions do not always list every ingredient. Inquire how gluten-free grains such as rice and risottos are cooked. Sometimes they are cooked in broth which may contain gluten. Confirm that separate, clean utensils and equipment will be used to prepare your meal.

Order simple, such as broiled fish with steamed vegetables and brown rice. Tell the waiter you want no sauce, no gravy, nothing added. Then, knowing your calorie objective, and that fish is about 50 Calories per ounce, most steamed vegetable servings average approximately 50 Calories per cup, and rice is about 100 Calories per ½ cup, decide how much to eat – and take the remainder home. And consider bringing your own gluten-free salad dressing to the restaurant.   If fresh fruit is not an option, pass on dessert and have the evening snack specified in the *90-Day Gluten-Free Smart Diet* meal plan for that day.

In a restaurant, most nutritionists recommend you eat the low-calorie items on your plate first. Start with the salad, soup and veggies. By the time you get to the chicken and starches you will hopefully be full enough to be content with smaller portions of the higher-calorie choices.

Day 41 - Recipe

Pasta e Fagioli

This is a variation of a traditional, nutritious peasant dish served in Italy.

14.5-oz can whole tomatoes with juice, crushed
14.5-oz can cannellini beans*, drained
1 cup of any tube-shaped GF pasta (page 222)
2 tablespoon olive oil
1 medium onion, diced
2 cloves garlic, minced
1 stalk celery, finely chopped
3 cups GF chicken stock (page 223)
2 cups fresh baby spinach or escarole
1 tsp dried basil
½ teaspoon dried oregano
2 Tbsp fresh parsley, chopped

Heat olive oil, onion and celery in large saucepan over medium heat. Sauté until onions are golden brown. Add garlic and stir constantly for one minute. Pour in tomatoes and their juices and bring to a boil. Add beans and GF chicken stock and return to a boil. Stir in spinach (or escarole) and seasonings. Simmer for about 5 minutes. Add pasta and cook about 15 minutes or until pasta is tender but firm. If needed, thin soup with hot water. Ladle into bowls. Garnish with grated GF cheese. **Serves 4**. About 300 Calories per serving.

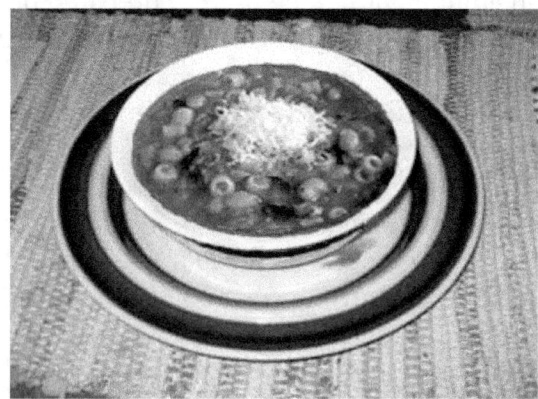

* Canned cannellini beans should be gluten free but check the ingredients on the container to be sure. Call the manufacturer and ask if the beans could contain trace gluten or could have been cross contaminated in their factory. Do not eat a food if you are not sure it is gluten free. Remember, if in doubt, go without.

Day 42 - Recipe

GF Blueberry Muffins

Wholesome blueberry muffins just like grandma used to make - but gluten free. Serve them at breakfast, or as a nutritious dessert, or a wonderful snack. (Make a dozen. Have one today and store the remainder in your freezer until they are called for again later in the diet.)

¼ cup sugar
¼ teaspoon vanilla
1¼ cups GF All Purpose flour (page 215)
2 teaspoons baking powder
¼ teaspoon salt
¾ cup blueberries (fresh or frozen)
2 eggs, beaten
½ cup milk
2 tablespoons vegetable oil

Preheat oven to 400 °F. Coat muffin tins with nonstick cooking spray. In a bowl combine dry ingredients. In another bowl combine wet ingredients and mix thoroughly. Add wet ingredients to dry ingredients and mix until just blended. Do not over mix. Gently fold in blueberries. Spoon batter into muffin tins until two-thirds full. Bake 15 minutes or until muffin tops are golden brown.

Yield is 12 Muffins, 125 Calories each

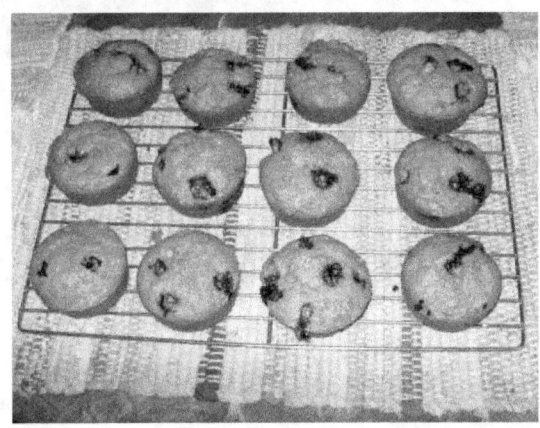

Diet Tip of the Day: **Acquire a good low-calorie cookbook**. Be sure the recipes cover breakfast, lunch and dinner, and all the recipes contain nutritional information, especially the calories per serving.

Day 43 - Recipe

Beef Kebob

  1 lb boneless beef tenderloin steaks, 1" thick
  8 ounces medium mushrooms
  2 medium bell peppers (any color), cut in pieces
Marinate ingredients: 2 tablespoons olive oil, 1 tablespoon chopped fresh oregano, 2 cloves garlic minced and ½ teaspoon ground black pepper

Cut beef steak into 1-inch square pieces. Combine marinate ingredients in large bowl. Add beef, mushrooms and bell pepper pieces. Toss to coat. Cover bowl and refrigerate for about two hours. Thread beef and vegetable pieces onto eight 12-inch metal skewers.

Grill kebobs over medium-high heat for 8 to 10 minutes, turning occasionally. Check center of meat with a small incision to determine when the meat is done.

Microwave a one-pound package of frozen mixed vegetables. Plate two kebob skewers and about one-quarter of the mixed veggies.
Serves 4. One plate consisting of two kebob skewers (350 Calories) plus ¼ pound of mixed green vegetables (40 Calories) totals about 390 Calories.

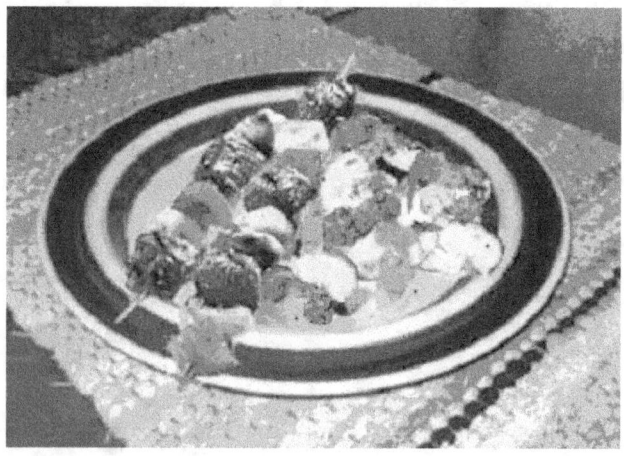

Diet Tip of the Day: Remember your stomach is about the size of your fist. So it doesn't take much food to fill it comfortably.

Day 44 - Recipe

Baked Haddock

  4 4-oz haddock fillets (or salmon fillets)
½ cup white wine (naturally gluten free)
½ cup GF non-fat yogurt mixed w ¼ cup pureed roasted red pepper
½ pound green beans
¾ pint cherry tomatoes (about 20)
1 tablespoon olive oil
¾ cup quinoa, prepared per package directions. (Note quinoa is naturally gluten free.)

Lightly dust fillets with flour. Dip in beaten egg white and then in GF Panko bread crumbs. Brown fillets in non-stick pan. Place fillets skin side down in baking dish coated with non-stick spray. Add white wine and cook in oven preheated to 350 °F for about 15 minutes. Spoon pan juices over fillets. Salt and pepper to taste.

Place green beans in skillet. Add ¼-inch of water and cook over medium heat until water boils off. Add cherry tomatoes and olive oil. Stir well and sauté for a few minutes. Season with fresh rosemary and oregano. Salt and pepper to taste.

Plate haddock fillet and spoon over yogurt-red pepper sauce. Garnish with fresh parsley. Add green beans & tomato mix and the quinoa. Serve hot.

Serves 4. One plate consisting of one haddock fillet (215 Calories) with green beans & tomato mix (65 Calories) and quinoa (120 Calories) totals 400 Calories.

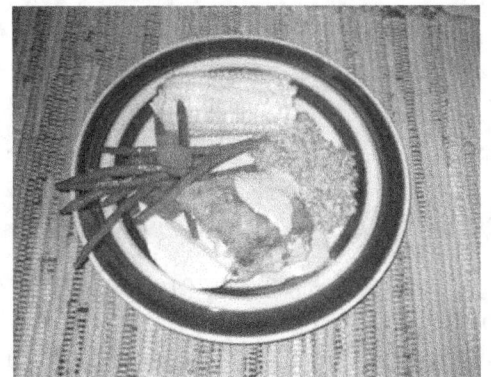

Corn-on-the-cob is only for the 1800 Calorie diet.

Day 45 - Recipe

Chicken Cacciatore

¾ lb skinless, boneless chicken breast halves
¼ lb of GF pasta
½ cup chopped onion
½ cup chopped green bell pepper
14.5-ounce can chopped tomatoes, drained
8-ounce can GF tomato sauce (page 217)
1½ teaspoons Italian seasoning (page 217)
⅓ cup sliced ripe olives
⅛ teaspoon black pepper
Cut chicken breasts into small pieces. Spray a large heavy skillet with olive oil flavored cooking spray.

Sauté chicken, onion and green pepper for 6 to 8 minutes. Stir in drained tomatoes and tomato sauce. Add Italian seasoning, olives and ⅛ teaspoon ground black pepper. Mix well to combine. Lower heat and simmer for 15 to 20 minutes, stirring occasionally.

Cook pasta per package directions. Ladle chicken and sauce over pasta and serve immediately.
Serves 4. About 310 Calories per serving

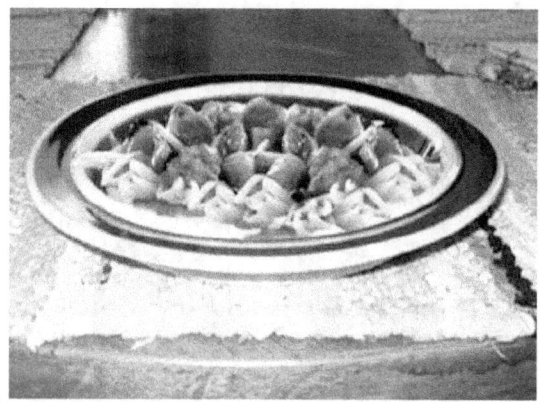

Diet Tip of the Day: Inevitably, you're going to be faced with a stressful situation. Instead of turning to food for comfort, be prepared with some non-food tactics that work for you, such as listening to music, reading, writing in a journal, or meditating.

Day 46 - Recipe

<u>Poached Cod in Tomato Broth</u>

2 cups dry white wine
1 cup clam juice*
2 cans (14.5-ounce) diced tomatoes, drained
1 small onion, diced
1 garlic clove, minced
½ tsp dried parsley, or sprigs of fresh parsley
1 bay leaf
12 black olives, pitted and halved
4 cod fish fillets (about 6 ounces each)
Note that sole, flounder, halibut or haddock may be substituted for cod.

Use a pan large enough to hold the fish in a single layer. Place all the ingredients except the fish in the pan. Over high heat, bring poaching liquid to a boil (pan uncovered). Reduce heat and simmer the liquid another 6 minutes.

Carefully place the fish filets in the liquid. Cover the pan and reduce heat until liquid is just simmering. Poach until fish are completely opaque and tender – about 8 minutes. Plate fish and ladle broth over fish.
<u>Serves 4</u>. 275 Calories per serving.

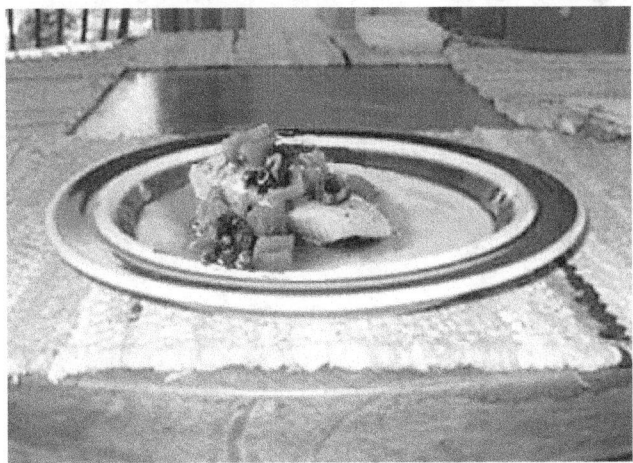

* Clam juice is naturally gluten free but check the label and with the manufacturer to make sure the facility used to process and package the clam juice is not also used to process gluten products.

Day 47 - Recipe

Chinese Dinner - Out

No recipe today. No cooking today. Have a Chinese dinner at your favorite restaurant, but make sure you choose a restaurant where you can eat gluten free and have a reasonable chance to achieve your calorie goal. For today, **your goal for dinner is a maximum of 640 Calories**. This includes any appetizer, soup, main course and any dessert.

Tips for Eating Chinese: Try bringing a restaurant card to the Chinese restaurant. The cards are available online and are designed to help explain a gluten-free diet to a waiter who might not speak English.

You can consume a lot of calories in a Chinese restaurant – if you order carelessly. For example a typical portion of General Tso's chicken is loaded with about 1,000 Calories, then add another 200 Calories for a cup of rice.

First rule, order simple. Rice noodles prepared with vegetables or chicken are generally a safe choice. Avoid brown sauce which may have a soy sauce base. Instead, ask for the dish to be prepared with a white sauce using corn starch. Then, knowing your 640 Calorie objective, and that chicken and fish are about 50 Calories per ounce, most steamed vegetable servings average approximately 50 Calories per cup, and rice is about 200 Calories per cup, decide how much of the meal you can eat – and take the remainder home. (Note that you will be eating half a serving of left over Chinese food for lunch tomorrow.) To stay within your maximum allowable calorie total, you should pass on dessert and have the evening snack (if any) specified for that day in the diet.

And although it is customary to share dishes at a Chinese restaurant, do not permit your dinner companions to contaminate your food. Make sure your friends do not use their gluten-contaminated spoons to serve food from your gluten-free dish.

Diet Tip of the Day: Inevitably, everyone on a diet hits a frustrating **weight-loss plateau**. Two ways to bust through the plateau are: first to reduce your calorie intake and second to step up your exercise intensity.

Day 48 - Recipe

Healthy Pasta Salad

½ pound GF fusilli pasta*, cooked until tender but firm
2 broccoli crowns, chopped
¼ pint cherry tomatoes (about 8), halved
½ cup black olives, halved
½ cup garbanzo beans (chick peas)**
½ cup fresh light mozzarella cheese (page 221), chopped
1 tablespoon basil
1 tablespoon rosemary
2 teaspoons garlic powder
¼ cup of a GF lite dressing (page 222)

Combine dry ingredients in a medium-size bowl. Stir in salad dressing.
Mix thoroughly. Salt and black pepper to taste.
Serves 4. 370 Calories per serving.

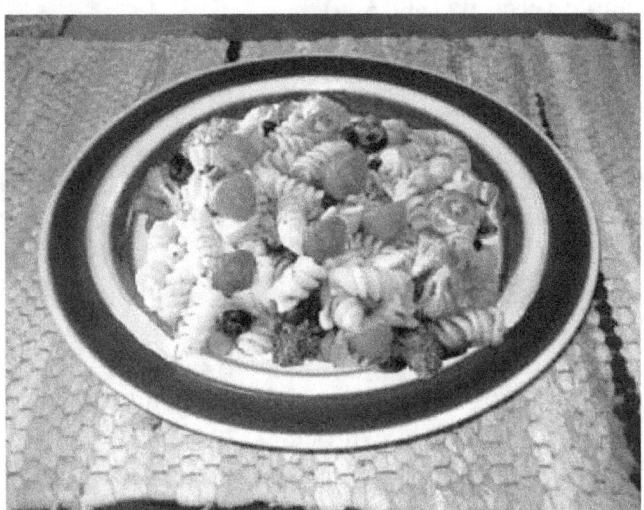

* We used Delallo Whole Grain Rice Fusilli. Chef, Gail Johnson said, "DeLallo pasta is very good with a springy bite and agreeable flavor." See page 222 for additional gluten-free pasta choices.

* Canned garbanzo beans should be gluten free but check the ingredients on the container to be sure. Call the manufacturer and ask if the beans could contain trace gluten or could have been cross contaminated in their factory. Do not eat a food if you are not sure it is gluten free. Remember, if in doubt, go without.

Day 49 - Recipe

Frozen Dinner

No recipe today. No cooking today. It's your day off! At this writing, Amy's and Artisan Bistro offer quite a few gluten-free frozen entrees. Smart Ones only makes two gluten-free entrees.

- Amy's Quinoa, Black Beans, Butternut Squash & Chard (**240 Cal**)
- Amy's Black Bean & Cheese Enchilada (**240 Cal**)
- Amy's Mushroom Risotto Bowl (**240 Cal**)
- Amy's Sweet & Sour Asian Noodle Bowl (**250 Cal**)
- Amy's Vegetable Parmesan Bowl (**260 Cal**)
- Amy's Brown Rice & Veggies Bowl – Light in Sodium (**260 Cal**)
- Amy's Brown Rice, Black-eyed Peas & Veggies Bowl (**290 Cal**)
- Amy's Teriyaki Bowl (**290 Cal**)
- Amy's Asian Noodle Stir Fry (**300 Cal**)
- Amy's Vegetable Lasagna (**300 Cal**)
- Amy's Thai Stir-Fry (**310 Cal**)
- Amy's Tofu Scramble (**320 Cal**)

- Artisan Bistro Wild Alaskan Salmon (**200 Cal**)
- Artisan Bistro Chicken Parmesan Bake (**200 Cal**)
- Artisan Bistro Turkey Cheddar Bake (**240 Cal**)
- Artisan Bistro Wild Alaskan Salmon Bake (**240 Cal**)
- Artisan Bistro Thai Style Yellow Curry with Chicken (**240 Cal**)
- Artisan Bistro Cheddar Beef Bake (**250 Cal**)
- Artisan Bistro Sesame Ginger with Salmon (**270 Cal**)
- Artisan Bistro Coconut Lemongrass with Chicken (**270 Cal**)
- Artisan Bistro Spiced Chicken Morocco (**270 Cal**)
- Artisan Bistro Albacore Tuna Bake (**280 Cal**)
- Artisan Bistro Thai Style Red Curry with Beef (**280 Cal**)
- Artisan Bistro Chicken Citron (**280 Cal**)
- Artisan Bistro Wild Alaskan Salmon with Pesto (**310 Cal**)
- Artisan Bistro Savory Turkey (**330 Cal**)
- Artisan Bistro Southwest Style Beef (**330 Cal**)
- Artisan Bistro Ginger Chicken (**350 Cal**)
- Artisan Bistro Beef with Mushroom Sauce (**350 Cal**)
- Artisan Bistro Wild Alaskan Salmon Cake (**370 Cal**)

- Smart Ones Lemon Herb Chicken Piccata (**250 Cal**)

- Smart Ones Santa Fe Style Rice & Beans (**290 Cal**)

And please read the important **Frozen-Food Safety Warning** in **Appendix D** (page 226).

<u>**Diet Tip of the Day:**</u> Experts agree that whether you are trying to lose weight or just maintain your weight, **it's calories that count**. It doesn't matter what foods the calories are from. To lose weight you must eat fewer calories than you burn. Calories count! Not carbs, not Weight Watchers points. Calories – period!

Day 50 - Recipe

Pan-Fried Sole

    4 sole fillets (6-ounces each), skinned
    1 tablespoon olive oil
    <u>Salsa Ingredients:</u>
    1 pint cherry tomatoes, quartered
    ¾ cup cucumber, finely chopped
    ⅓ cup yellow bell pepper, finely chopped
    3 tablespoons fresh basil, chopped
    2 tablespoons capers
    1½ tablespoons shallots, finely chopped
    1 tablespoon balsamic vinegar
    2 teaspoons lemon rind, grated

Combine salsa ingredients in a bowl and stir in ½ teaspoon salt and ⅛ teaspoon black pepper. Mix thoroughly.

Heat olive oil in a large nonstick skillet over medium-high heat. Season sole fillets with
½ teaspoon salt and ⅛ teaspoon black pepper. Add fish to pan; cook about 1½ minutes on each side or until fish flakes easily when tested with a fork. Spoon salsa over fish and serve immediately.
<u>Serves 4</u>. 325 Calories per serving

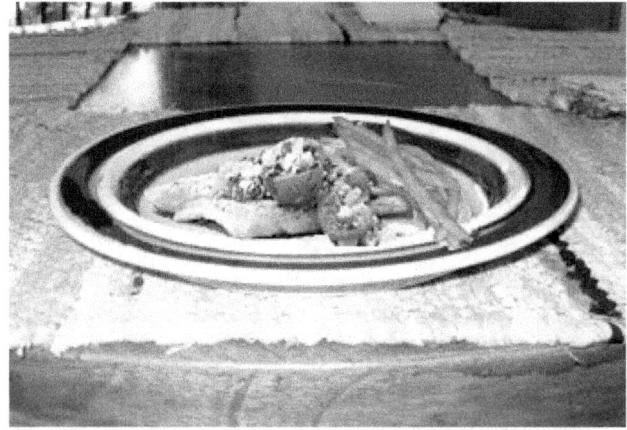

<u>Diet Tip of the Day:</u> If you are overweight start on a weight loss diet now because it will only become **more difficult to lose weight as you get older**.

Day 51 - Recipe

<u>Beans & Greens Salad</u> (Repeated)

⅓ cup chopped oregano
⅓ cup chopped parsley
3 cloves garlic, chopped
1 lemon, juiced

Prepare dressing by combining above ingredients and stirring in ¼ cup extra-virgin olive oil. Salt and pepper to taste.

½ pound mesclun mix (mixed greens)
¼ pound green beans
19-ounce can garbanzo beans (chickpeas)*

Arrange mesclun mix, garbanzo beans and green beans on a large platter. Drizzle dressing over beans and greens.
<u>Serves 4</u>. Approximately 260 Calories per serving.

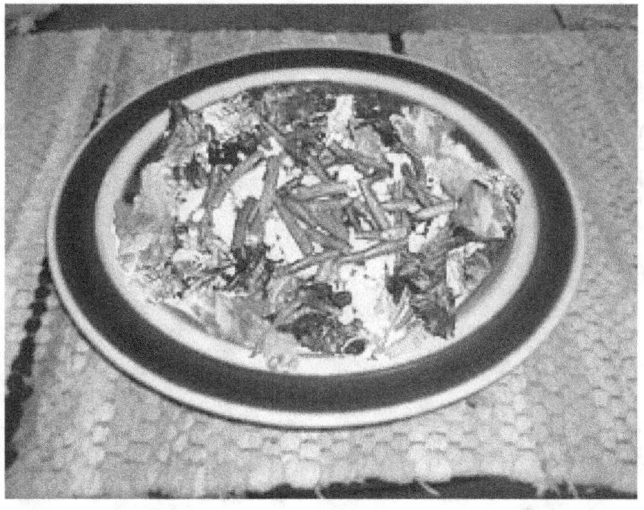

* Canned garbanzo beans should be gluten free but check the ingredients on the container to be sure. Call the manufacturer and ask if the beans could contain trace gluten or could have been cross contaminated in their factory. Do not eat a food if you are not sure it is gluten free. Remember, if in doubt, go without.

<u>Diet Tip of the Day:</u> **Fat-free isn't always your best bet**. Low fat doesn't necessarily mean low calorie! Most often sugar is substituted for fat and the calorie total remains the same or even higher. Instead, look for low-calorie or reduced-calorie foods.

Day 52 - Recipe

Chicken Piccata

1 pound boneless skinless chicken breast halves
2 teaspoons olive oil
1 teaspoon minced garlic
¼ cup shallots, diced
¾ pound fresh green beans, washed and snipped
1 teaspoon lemon juice
¼ cup capers, rinsed
2 fresh lemons, cut into small wedges

In a skillet, heat olive oil and minced garlic over medium heat. Sauté chicken breasts and shallots for two to three minutes, tossing often, until chicken is partially cooked. Add green beans and one teaspoon of lemon juice and sauté for an additional two to three minutes, or until chicken is completely cooked and green beans are al dente. Add capers; and cover chicken. Let sit for one more minute to warm capers. Serve immediately with wedges of lemon.

Serves 4. 270 calories per serving

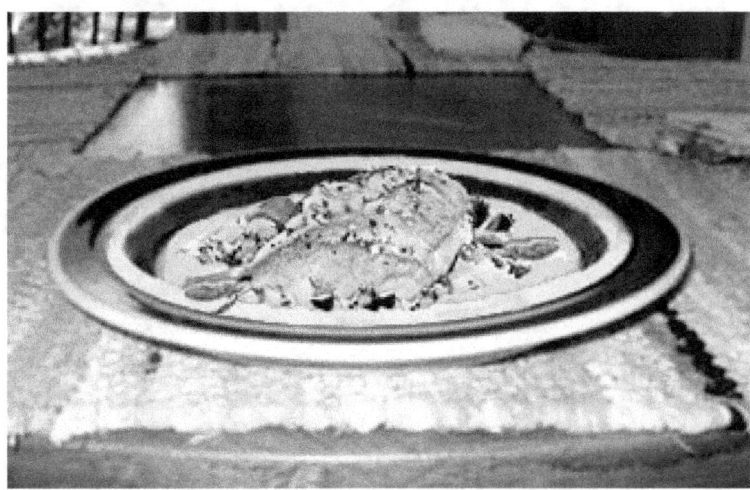

Diet Tip of the Day: Handle **occasional overeating by compensating**. To do this, estimate how far you have strayed from your weight-loss diet and then make amends at the next opportunity (usually the next meal or two) – by eating less.

Day 53 - Recipe

<u>Beef Steak Strips</u>

   1 lb top loin sirloin, or top round about ¾" thick
   1 tsp garlic, finely chopped
   ½ tsp dry thyme
   ½ tsp salt and ¼ tsp black peppercorns
Cut the steak into 3-inch long by ¼-inch thick strips Sprinkle the beef strips with garlic, thyme, salt and pepper. Prepare a large non-stick skillet over medium-high heat. Add the steak strips and shake the skillet constantly to avoid sticking. Cook approximately 2 to 3 minutes until meat is seared but pink inside. Check the center by making small incision.
<u>Serves 4</u>. About 330 Calories per serving (meat only).

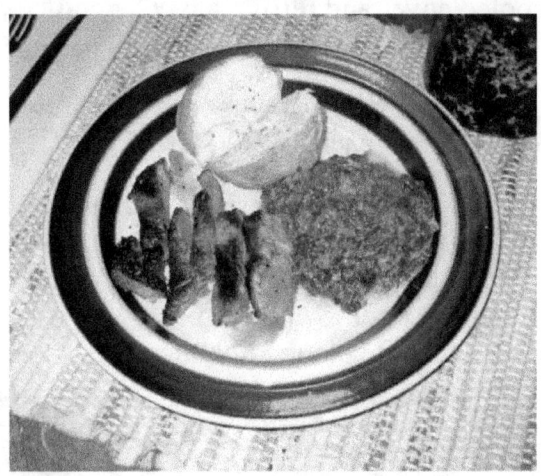

<u>Diet Tip of the Day:</u> Bear in mind, that knowledge and the discipline to **workout regularly** are far more important than fancy equipment.

Day 54 - Recipe

Tina's Grilled Scallops & Polenta

1 pound sea scallops
¾ cup GF polenta (page 216) cornmeal
¾ cup skim milk
1 medium Portobello mushroom
½ pound green beans
¼ cup chopped red onion
16 asparagus spear
1 teaspoon extra-virgin olive oil

Bring 1½ cups of water and skim milk to rapid boil. Add salt to taste. Slowly add polenta while stirring. Reduce heat. Continue stirring until desired consistency is reached. Pour polenta into lightly greased pan. After polenta has cooled cover and refrigerate. Cut chilled polenta into 4 pieces. Grill on medium-hot fire – about two minutes on each side.

Brush Portobello mushroom and asparagus spear with olive oil and place on grill for about 3 minutes on each side.

Grill scallops on medium-hot fire. Turn after two minutes or when first side turns opaque. Grill until second side turns opaque – about another 2 minutes. Don't overcook but test a scallop by cutting to make sure it's cooked through. Salt and pepper to taste.

Serves 4. The food on the plate pictured below totals about 380 Calories.

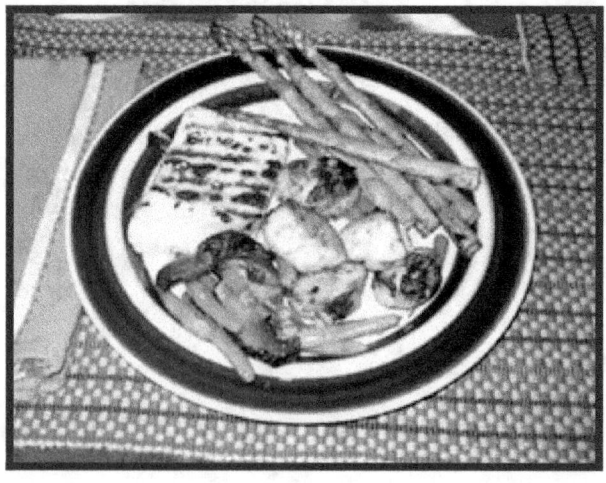

Day 55 - Recipe

Hearty Vegetable Soup

  2 15-oz cans white kidney beans*, drained
  1 tablespoon olive oil
  ½ large yellow onion, chopped
  2 garlic cloves, minced
  1 cup chopped fresh tomatoes
  2 celery stalks, cut into ½-inch pieces
  1½ carrots, cut into ½-inch pieces
  5 cups GF vegetable stock (page 223)
  1 medium potato, cut into ½-inch pieces
  ¼ cup chopped fresh basil
  ¼ head of red cabbage, cut into ½-inch pieces
  2 zucchini or summer squash, cut into ½-inch pieces

Heat olive oil in a large pot over medium heat. Add onion and garlic.
Sauté 5 minutes. Add green cabbage, tomatoes, celery, and carrots.
Sauté 10 minutes. Add beans, 5 cups of stock, potatoes, and basil. Bring
to a boil. Reduce heat, cover and simmer for one hour. Add red
cabbage, zucchini and salt . Cover and simmer until vegetables are
tender, about 20 minutes longer. Stir in about ¼ cup Parmesan cheese
and sprinkle a dash of Tabasco hot sauce if you want a little zip.
Serves 4. 360 Calories per serving

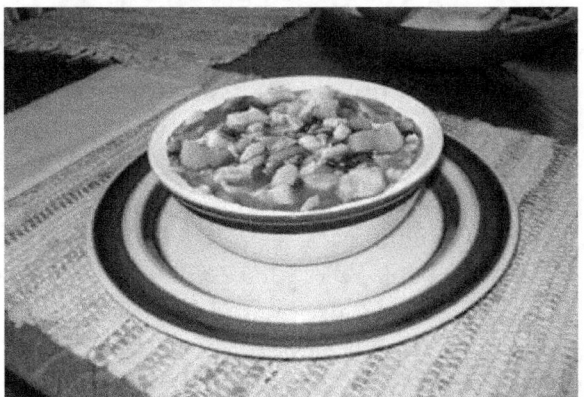

* Canned white kidney beans should be gluten free but check the ingredients on the
container to be sure. Call the manufacturer and ask if the beans could contain trace
gluten or could have been cross contaminated in their factory. Do not eat a food if you
are not sure it is gluten free. Remember, if in doubt, go without.

Day 56 - Recipe

<u>Frozen Dinner</u>

No recipe today. No cooking today. It's your day off! At this writing, Amy's and Artisan Bistro offer quite a few gluten-free frozen entrees. Smart Ones only makes two gluten-free entrees. Glutino also makes two gluten-free frozen entrees, but each contain 400 Calories, and are not included in the following list.

- Amy's Quinoa, Black Beans, Butternut Squash & Chard (**240 Cal**)
- Amy's Black Bean & Cheese Enchilada (**240 Cal**)
- Amy's Mushroom Risotto Bowl (**240 Cal**)
- Amy's Sweet & Sour Asian Noodle Bowl (**250 Cal**)
- Amy's Vegetable Parmesan Bowl (**260 Cal**)
- Amy's Brown Rice & Veggies Bowl – Light in Sodium (**260 Cal**)
- Amy's Brown Rice, Black-eyed Peas & Veggies Bowl (**290 Cal**)
- Amy's Teriyaki Bowl (**290 Cal**)
- Amy's Asian Noodle Stir Fry (**300 Cal**)
- Amy's Vegetable Lasagna (**300 Cal**)
- Amy's Thai Stir-Fry (**310 Cal**)
- Amy's Tofu Scramble (**320 Cal**)

- Artisan Bistro Wild Alaskan Salmon (**200 Cal**)
- Artisan Bistro Chicken Parmesan Bake (**200 Cal**)
- Artisan Bistro Turkey Cheddar Bake (**240 Cal**)
- Artisan Bistro Wild Alaskan Salmon Bake (**240 Cal**)
- Artisan Bistro Thai Style Yellow Curry with Chicken (**240 Cal**)
- Artisan Bistro Cheddar Beef Bake (**250 Cal**)
- Artisan Bistro Sesame Ginger with Salmon (**270 Cal**)
- Artisan Bistro Coconut Lemongrass with Chicken (**270 Cal**)
- Artisan Bistro Spiced Chicken Morocco (**270 Cal**)
- Artisan Bistro Albacore Tuna Bake (**280 Cal**)
- Artisan Bistro Thai Style Red Curry with Beef (**280 Cal**)
- Artisan Bistro Chicken Citron (**280 Cal**)
- Artisan Bistro Wild Alaskan Salmon with Pesto (**310 Cal**)
- Artisan Bistro Savory Turkey (**330 Cal**)
- Artisan Bistro Southwest Style Beef (**330 Cal**)
- Artisan Bistro Ginger Chicken (**350 Cal**)
- Artisan Bistro Beef with Mushroom Sauce (**350 Cal**)
- Artisan Bistro Wild Alaskan Salmon Cake (**370 Cal**)

- Smart Ones Lemon Herb Chicken Piccata (**250 Cal**)
- Smart Ones Santa Fe Style Rice & Beans (**290 Cal**)

Also note that **340 Calories are allocated for this meal**. But almost all of the above have less than 340 Calories. Use the excess calories anyway you wish. Splurge on extra dessert or save the calories for another day!

And please read the important **Frozen-Food Safety Warning** in **Appendix D** (page 226).

<u>**Diet Tip of the Day**</u>: To prevent or delay the onset of type II diabetes, experts urge the overweight to lose weight and work out regularly. Weight loss helps your body use insulin more efficiently, and exercise helps metabolize excess circulating blood glucose.

Day 57 - Recipe

Salmon with Mango Salsa

 4 salmon fillets (about 5 ounces each)
 1½ pounds baby new potatoes, halved
 1 mango, ripe
 3 green onions, finely chopped
 3 tablespoons chopped fresh cilantro
 2 tablespoons lemon juice
 2 teaspoons extra-virgin olive oil
 4 cups watercress

Remove any tiny bones from salmon. Press crushed peppercorns into flesh side of salmon. Set aside. Place halved potatoes into saucepan. Cover with water and bring to a boil. Reduce the heat and simmer until tender, about 10-12 minutes and drain.

Prepare salsa: Peel and seed the mango. Dice the mango flesh and put into a large bowl. Mix in green onions, cilantro, lemon juice, olive oil, and an optional dash of Tabasco*.

Heat a grill pan coated with nonstick cooking spray over medium-high heat. Place salmon fillets in pan, skin-side down. Cook for 4 minutes. Turn fish over and cook until done, about another 4 minutes. Arrange watercress and new potatoes on serving plates. Place salmon on top and spoon over mango salsa.
Serves 4. 460 Calories per serving

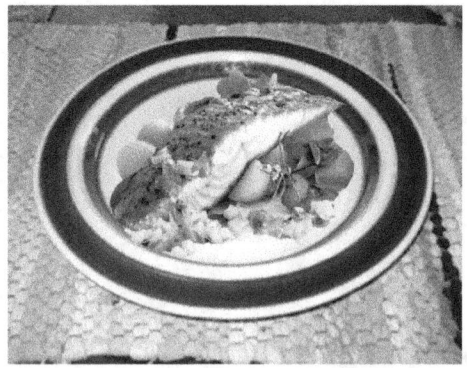

* Testing has not detected gluten in Tabasco products. But be wary because Tabasco is derived from grains and its gluten-free is not a certainty.

Day 58 - Recipe

<u>Pork Chop with Orange Slices</u>

4   loin pork chops, ½-inch-thick (about 1½ lbs total, bones included)
8   orange slices, ¼-inch-thick
1   teaspoon salt
¾   teaspoon black pepper
¼   cup orange marmalade preserve
½   cup bottled GF fruit-based barbecue sauce

<u>Marinade</u>: ½ cup orange juice, 2 teaspoons GF soy sauce (page 217) and ¼ teaspoon crushed red pepper.

Combine pork chops and marinade in large re-sealable plastic bag. Refrigerate for about 30 minutes. Remove chops from marinade and season with salt and black pepper.

Stir together orange marmalade and BBQ sauce in a small bowl. Brush one side of pork chops evenly with half of marmalade-BBQ mixture. Grill chops, with marmalade-BBQ mixture side up over medium-high heat (about 375°) for about 5 minutes or until done. Turn chops, and brush with remaining marmalade-BBQ mixture. Grill another 5 minutes or until done. Grill orange slices over medium-high heat, 1 minute on each side.
<u>Serves 4</u>. 470 Calories per serving (includes pork chop and two orange slices)

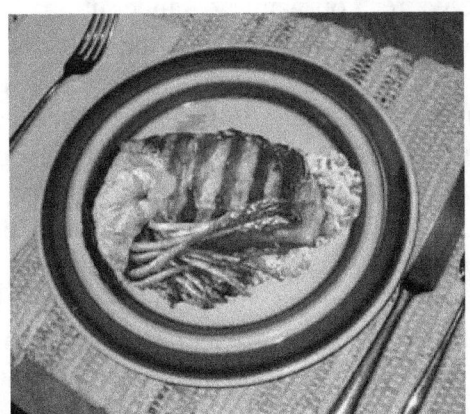

* Such as Grandville's Gourmet GF Pineapple BBQ Jam

Day 59 - Recipe

Fish Dinner - Out

No recipe today. No cooking today. Have a fish dinner at a restaurant, but make sure you choose a restaurant where you have a good chance to eat gluten free and achieve your calorie goal. For today, your **goal for dinner is a maximum of 595 Calories**. This includes appetizer, soup, main course and dessert.

Tips for Eating Fish Out: The following is almost an exact repeat of the advice given eating out on previous days. First make sure you choose a restaurant where gluten-free food is available and where you have a good chance to achieve your calorie goal. Before you out go read the menu online and reduce your food choices so you can have more focused questions for the staff. You are more likely to get a safe meal if you call the restaurant before you go to let them know of your gluten-free needs. And call during a slow time so you can have the host's complete attention.

In the restaurant, to ensure you are served a gluten-free meal, it is important to communicate your need to eat 100 percent gluten-free assertively but pleasantly. Try to speak directly to the chef or manager. Otherwise, ask your server what is in the food and how it is prepared. Menu descriptions do not always list every ingredient. Inquire how gluten-free grains such as rice and risottos are cooked. Sometimes they are cooked in broth which may contain gluten. Confirm that separate, clean utensils and equipment will be used to prepare your meal.

Order simple, such as broiled fish with steamed vegetables and brown rice. Tell the waiter you want no sauce, no gravy, nothing added. Then, knowing your calorie objective, and that fish is about 50 Calories per ounce, most steamed vegetable servings average approximately 50 Calories per cup, and rice is about 100 Calories per ½ cup, decide how much to eat – and take the remainder home. And consider bringing your own gluten-free salad dressing to the restaurant. If fresh fruit is not an option, pass on dessert and have the evening snack specified in the *90-Day Gluten-Free Smart Diet* meal plan for that day.

In a restaurant, most nutritionists recommend you eat the low-calorie items on your plate first. Start with the salad, soup and veggies. By the time you get to the chicken and starches you will hopefully be full enough to be content with smaller portions of the higher-calorie choices.

Day 60 - Recipe

<u>Chicken Stew over Rice</u>

4	boneless skinless chicken breasts (about 1 lb)
1	medium Onion
3	stalks celery
12	mushrooms
2	cups baby carrots
3	cups broccoli florets
½	teaspoon black pepper
¼	teaspoon herb seasoning (page 217) blend
2	teaspoons Worcestershire Sauce (page 218)
1	bay leaf
½	cup Amy's Cream of Tomato Soup
½	cup 2% milk
1	tablespoon GF all-purpose flour (page 215)

Prepare a large, heavy, stove-top pot with GF cooking spray. Sauté at medium-high heat finely chop onion until caramelized. Cut chicken into bite size pieces and add to pot. Cook and toss until chicken is no longer pink. Add black pepper, herb seasoning and Worcestershire sauce. Stir. Add sliced celery and mushrooms, and then broccoli, carrots and bay leaf. Pour in Cream of Tomato soup, milk and flour. Gradually add one cup water while stirring. (You may want to add more water to get consistency desired.) Simmer until hot and flavors have combined. Serve over rice.

<u>Serves 4</u>. 360 Calories per serving (not including the brown rice below the stew).

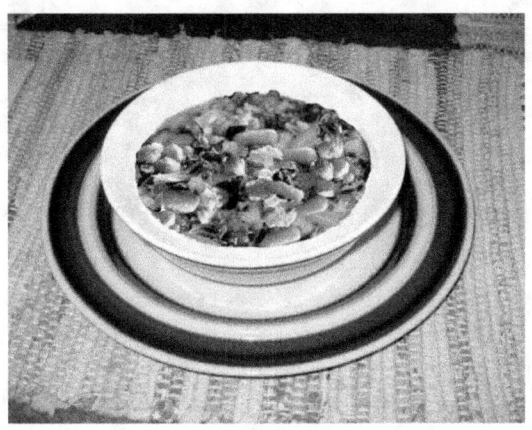

Day 61 - Recipe

Shrimp over Spaghetti

½ lb GF spaghetti
1 lb shrimp, peeled and de-veined
6 ounces dry white wine
3 tablespoons olive oil
3 cloves garlic, sliced thin
¼ cup chopped basil leaves

Cook spaghetti according to package directions. Save ½ cup of the pasta cooking water.

In a large skillet over medium heat, cook olive oil and garlic, stirring until garlic turns golden, and then discard garlic. Add shrimp and increase heat to medium-high and stir in chopped basil leaves, white wine and ½ cup cooking water. Cook another 2 to 3 minutes or until shrimp are just firm. Spoon shrimp and sauce over spaghetti. Season with salt and black pepper. Garnish with parsley.

Serves 4. 450 Calories per serving

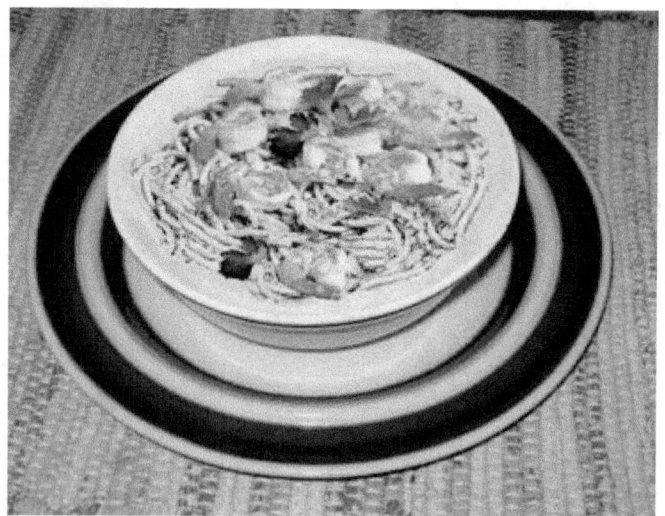

Diet Tip of the Day: If your caloric intake on a weight-loss diet is constant, your **rate of weight loss will decrease with time**. So if you want to lose weight at a constant rate over time, you must eat slightly less (or exercise harder) as you lose weight.

Day 62 - Recipe

<u>Beef Burgundy</u>

    1 lb boneless beef chuck, trimmed & cut in 1" pieces
    2 large carrots, cut into 1-inch pieces
    1 medium onion, cut into 1-inch pieces
    1 tablespoon GF all-purpose flour (page 215)
    1 tablespoon Hunt's GF tomato paste
    1 clove garlic, crushed
    1 tablespoon olive oil
    1 cup dry red wine
    2 sprigs fresh thyme
    10 ounces mushrooms, sliced in half
    8 ounces frozen peas

In Dutch oven, heat oil on medium-high until hot. Add beef and cook 5 to 6 minutes or until beef is browned on all sides. Transfer beef to a bowl. Preheat oven to 325° F. To drippings in Dutch oven, add carrots, garlic, and onion. Stir occasionally and cook 10 minutes or until vegetables are browned and tender. Stir in flour, tomato paste, ½ teaspoon salt, and ¼ teaspoon black pepper, and cook another minute. Add wine and heat to boiling, stirring until browned bits are loosened from bottom of Dutch oven. Return meat and any juices in the bowl to Dutch oven. Add thyme and mushrooms; bring to a boil. Cover and bake 1½ hours or until meat is fork-tender. Discard thyme sprigs. Before stew is done, cook peas per package instructions and add peas to Dutch oven.
Serves 4. 350 Calories per serving

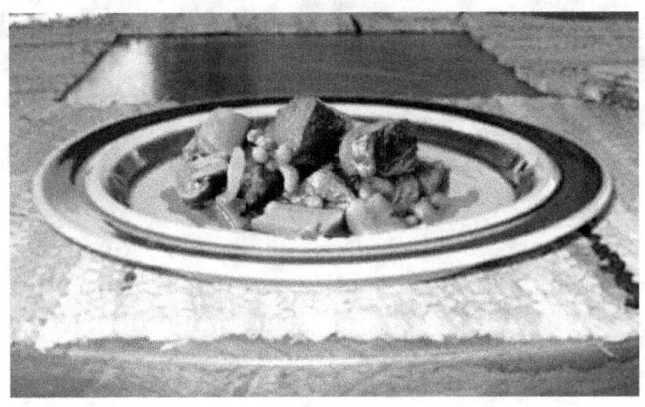

Day 63 - Recipe

Chicken Cutlet

Buy 4 skinless, boneless chicken cutlets or breast halves (about 1 lb), flattened to about ¼ to ½-inch thick.

    ¾ cup GF Panko bread crumbs (page 216)
    ⅓ cup grated Parmesan cheese
    1 egg, beaten
    4 tablespoons extra-virgin olive oil, divided

Season chicken cutlets with salt and pepper. Combine bread crumbs and Parmesan cheese in a shallow bowl. Whisk egg in a separate shallow bowl. Dip chicken in egg and then coat both sides in crumb mixture.

Heat 2 tablespoons of olive oil in large skillet over medium-high heat. Add 2 cutlets, and cook 2 minutes on each side or until cooked through. Repeat with 2 tablespoons olive oil and remaining 2 cutlets. Serve hot. **Serves 4.** 450 Calories per serving (chicken cutlet only)

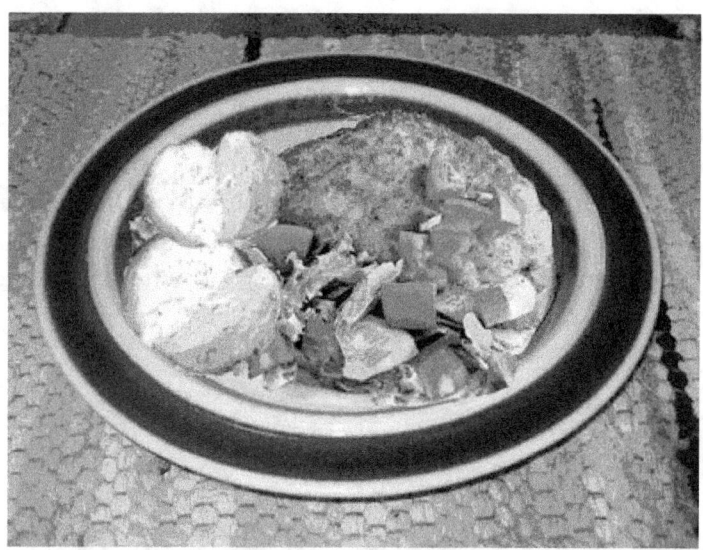

Diet Tip of the Day: **Working out at home** has some significant advantages. Your workout takes less time because you don't have to drive back and forth to a fitness facility; and you have the flexibility of dividing your workout into small time segments to fit your day, and of course working out at home is less expensive.

Day 64 - Recipe

Personal-Size Meat Loaf

1 pound extra lean ground beef
⅓ cup quick oats
2 egg whites
½ cup chipotle salsa (page 217), divided
¼ cup ketchup, divided

Place egg whites in a large bowl, mixing well with a whisk. Stir in oats, 6 tablespoons salsa, and 2 tablespoons ketchup. Add beef and mix well. Divide beef mixture into 4 equal portions, shaping each into an oval-shaped loaf. and place loaves on baking pan lined with tin foil and coated with cooking spray. Bake in preheated oven at 350°F for 30 minutes or until done.

Combine remaining 2 tablespoons salsa and 2 tablespoons ketchup in a small bowl. Spread mixture evenly over individual meat loaves.
Serves 4. 410 Calories per serving (meat loaf only)

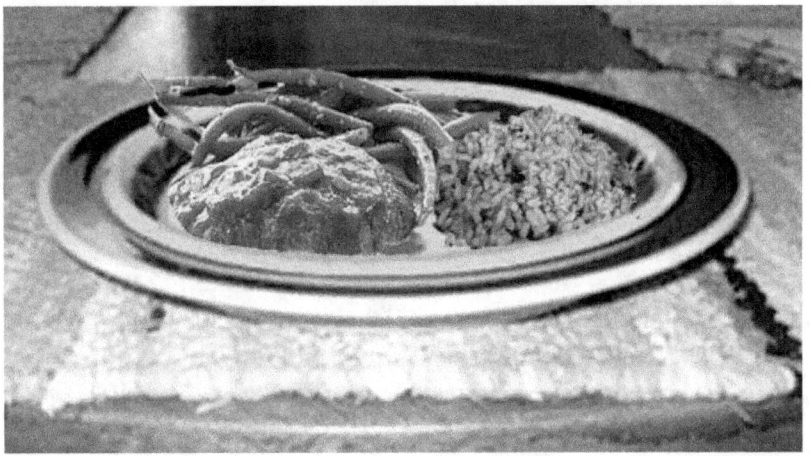

Diet Tip of the Day: To make sure you stay on track, **weigh in once a week**. There may be times when you might not see a weight loss, often because lost fat is temporarily replaced by water. This condition will gradually be corrected as you continue dieting.

Day 65 - Recipe

Frozen Dinner

No recipe today. No cooking today. It's your day off! At this writing, Amy's and Artisan Bistro offer quite a few gluten-free frozen entrees. Smart Ones only makes two gluten-free entrees. Glutino also makes two gluten-free frozen entrees, but each contain 400 Calories, and are not included in the following list.

- Amy's Quinoa, Black Beans, Butternut Squash & Chard (**240 Cal**)
- Amy's Black Bean & Cheese Enchilada (**240 Cal**)
- Amy's Mushroom Risotto Bowl (**240 Cal**)
- Amy's Sweet & Sour Asian Noodle Bowl (**250 Cal**)
- Amy's Vegetable Parmesan Bowl (**260 Cal**)
- Amy's Brown Rice & Veggies Bowl – Light in Sodium (**260 Cal**)
- Amy's Brown Rice, Black-eyed Peas & Veggies Bowl (**290 Cal**)
- Amy's Teriyaki Bowl (**290 Cal**)
- Amy's Asian Noodle Stir Fry (**300 Cal**)
- Amy's Vegetable Lasagna (**300 Cal**)
- Amy's Thai Stir-Fry (**310 Cal**)
- Amy's Tofu Scramble (**320 Cal**)

- Artisan Bistro Wild Alaskan Salmon (**200 Cal**)
- Artisan Bistro Chicken Parmesan Bake (**200 Cal**)
- Artisan Bistro Turkey Cheddar Bake (**240 Cal**)
- Artisan Bistro Wild Alaskan Salmon Bake (**240 Cal**)
- Artisan Bistro Thai Style Yellow Curry with Chicken (**240 Cal**)
- Artisan Bistro Cheddar Beef Bake (**250 Cal**)
- Artisan Bistro Sesame Ginger with Salmon (**270 Cal**)
- Artisan Bistro Coconut Lemongrass with Chicken (**270 Cal**)
- Artisan Bistro Spiced Chicken Morocco (**270 Cal**)
- Artisan Bistro Albacore Tuna Bake (**280 Cal**)
- Artisan Bistro Thai Style Red Curry with Beef (**280 Cal**)
- Artisan Bistro Chicken Citron (**280 Cal**)
- Artisan Bistro Wild Alaskan Salmon with Pesto (**310 Cal**)
- Artisan Bistro Savory Turkey (**330 Cal**)
- Artisan Bistro Southwest Style Beef (**330 Cal**)
- Artisan Bistro Ginger Chicken (**350 Cal**)
- Artisan Bistro Beef with Mushroom Sauce (**350 Cal**)
- Artisan Bistro Wild Alaskan Salmon Cake (**370 Cal**)

- Smart Ones Lemon Herb Chicken Piccata (**250 Cal**)
- Smart Ones Santa Fe Style Rice & Beans (**290 Cal**)

Please read the important **Frozen-Food Safety Warning** in **Appendix D** (page 226).

Diet Tip of the Day: **Muscle** is active tissue, fat is not. The more muscle you have, the more calories you burn. Muscle uses a significant number of calories every day for repair and rebuilding, giving your metabolism a boost even when you're resting. So make sure strengthening exercises (like weight lifting) are part of your workout.

Pepper & Mushroom Pizza

2 9-inch diameter GF pizza crust*
1 large red pepper, sliced
6 medium mushrooms, sliced
1 medium onion, sliced
3 ounces part-skim shredded mozzarella cheese
2 cups GF tomato sauce (page 217)
1 tablespoon olive oil, divided

Over medium high heat, sauté onion in two teaspoons of olive oil. Add pepper slices, onion slices and mushroom slices and cook until they softened.

Brush one side of pizza crust with remaining olive oil. Spread tomato sauce on crust. Arrange pepper, onion and mushroom slices and sprinkle shredded mozzarella cheese on top.

In oven preheated to 375°F, place pizza on baking tin coated with cooking spray. Cook approximately 10 minutes or until cheese melts and bottom of crust turns brown.

Serves 4. 265 Calories per serving

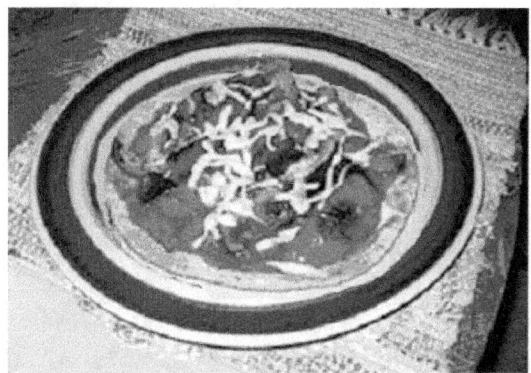

* We used Udi's Pizza Crust - 8 oz pkg which contains two 9-inch pizza crusts.

Diet Tip of the Day: On a reducing diet, **when you lose – you win**! You win a much better chance for a longer healthier life, you win a sense of well-being, you win a more attractive appearance – and finally you win a feeling of accomplishment.

Day 67 - Recipe

Chicken Dinner - Out

No recipe today. No cooking today. Today you eat at a restaurant. But when you are on a gluten-free reducing diet, eating in a restaurant can be a double challenge. First, most restaurant portions are huge, easily totaling more than 1,000 Calories, and then many restaurants do not offer gluten-free menu selections. On the *90-Day Gluten-Free Smart Diet*, a dinner type (i.e., fish, chicken, etc) and a calorie target are specified. For example Day 7 of the 1,200 Calorie diet calls for a chicken dinner and allows you 530 Calories for appetizer, soup, main course and dessert. Follow these tips to make sure your dinning experience is low calorie, gluten-free and pleasant.

Make sure you choose a restaurant where gluten-free food is available and where you have a fighting chance to achieve your calorie goal. Before you out go read the menu online and reduce your food choices so you can have more focused questions for the staff. You are more likely to get a safe meal if you call the restaurant before you go to let them know of your gluten-free needs. And call during a slow time so you can have the host's complete attention.

In the restaurant, to ensure you are served a gluten-free meal, it is important to communicate your need to eat 100 percent gluten-free assertively but amiably. Try to speak directly to the chef or manager. Otherwise, ask your server what is in the food and how it is prepared. Menu descriptions do not always list every ingredient. Inquire how gluten-free grains such as rice and risottos are cooked. Sometimes they are cooked in broth which may contain gluten. Confirm that separate, clean utensils and equipment will be used to prepare your meal.

Order something simple, such as skinless white meat broiled chicken breast with steamed vegetables and brown rice. Tell the waiter you want no sauce, no gravy, nothing added. Then, knowing your calorie objective, and that most fish and chicken are about 50 Calories per ounce, most steamed vegetable servings average approximately 50 Calories per cup, and rice is about 100 Calories per ½ cup, decide how much to eat – and take the remainder home. And consider bringing your own gluten-free salad dressing to the restaurant. If fresh fruit is not an option, pass on dessert and have the evening snack specified in the *90-Day Gluten-Free Smart Diet* meal plan for that day.

In a restaurant, most nutritionists recommend you eat the low-calorie items on your plate first. Start with the salad, soup and veggies. By the time you get to the chicken and starches you will hopefully be full enough to be content with smaller portions of the higher-calorie choices. (Incidentally, feel free to substitute skinless white meat turkey for chicken.)

Diet Tip of the Day: When you're eating out, consider **ordering children's portions** or a small sandwich as a way to trim calories and get the size of your meals under control.

Day 68 - Recipe

Pork Medallions in Lime Sauce

1 pound pork tenderloin
⅓ cup GF all purpose flour (page 215)
2 tablespoons olive oil
1 tablespoon unsalted butter
½ cup of white wine
¼ cup lime juice
2 stalks celery, chopped
1 medium onion, chopped

Trim away the thin silver skin on the tenderloin and all visible fat. Discard trimmings. Cut tenderloin into ½ to ¾ inch thick medallions. Sprinkle medallions with salt and pepper. Place flour in a shallow dish and coat pork medallions. Warm olive oil in a large skillet over medium-low heat. Working in batches if necessary, cook pork medallions, turning once, until well browned on both sides, about 5 minutes total. (Note internal pork temperature should be 160° F.) Transfer pork to a plate.

Add the wine and lime juice to skillet and bring to boil, scraping up browned bits from bottom of pan with wooden spoon and stirring occasionally, until thickened, about 4 minutes. Remove from heat; stir in butter, chopped celery and onion. Return pork to pan and warm though, turning medallions to coat with sauce.

Serves 4. 450 Calories per serving (pork medallions and sauce only)

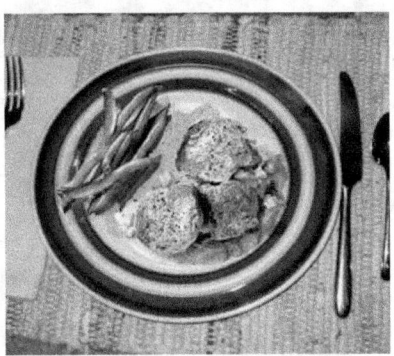

Diet Tip of the Day: Protein and carbohydrates are about 4 Calories per gram (110 Calories per ounce) and fat is 9 Calories per gram (260 Calories per ounce).

Day 69 - Recipe

Healthy Chicken Salad

4	skinless, boneless chicken breast halves, cooked
2	beefsteak tomatoes, cut into large pieces
1	celery heart, chopped
¼	pound roasted red peppers, from jar, chopped
1	small red onion, peeled, halved
10	black olives, halved
1	small bunch basil, leaves only
1½	tablespoons balsamic vinegar
4	tablespoons extra-virgin olive oil, divided
4	slices GF bread cut into 1-inch squares

Croutons: Toss GF croutons (bread squares) in ½ tablespoon olive oil.
Combine spices: oregano, parsley, garlic powder, salt and black pepper.
Sprinkle spice mix on croutons and then place them on foil-lined baking
pan. Bake 10 minutes at 350° F. Turn croutons and bake another 5
minutes.

Shred cooked chicken and mix with croutons, tomatoes, celery, roasted
peppers, red onion, olives and basil in large bowl and season with salt
and black pepper. Drizzle with 3 tablespoons extra-virgin olive oil and
1½ tablespoons balsamic vinegar and toss.
Serves 4. 330 Calories per serving

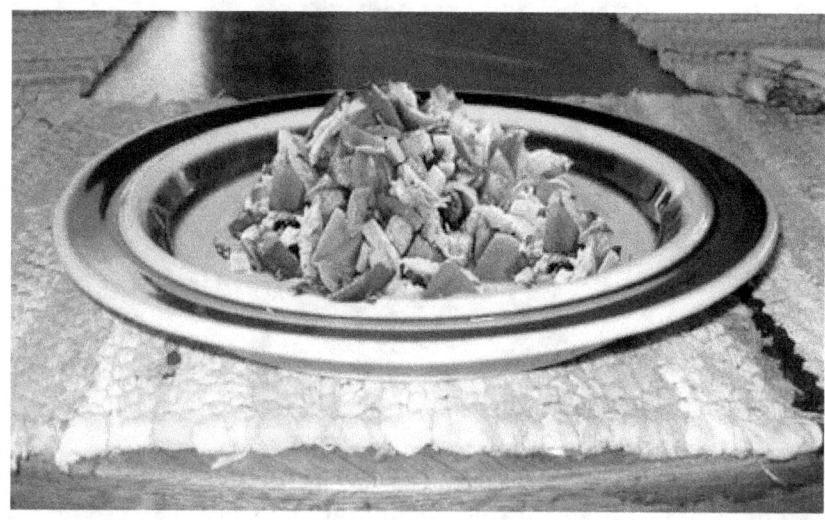

Day 70 - Recipe

<u>Baked Cod</u>

4   cod fish fillets (4 to 5 ounces each)
2   tablespoons GF all purpose flour (page 215)
2   tablespoons GF cornmeal (page 215)
2   tablespoons minced fresh herbs
2   teaspoons lemon juice

Sprinkle cod with lemon juice. Mix flour, cornmeal and herbs and dust the cod with the cornmeal-herb mixture. Bake in oven at 375 °F for 10 minutes. Add salt and black pepper to taste.

<u>Serves 4</u>. One serving is 230 Calories (cod only).

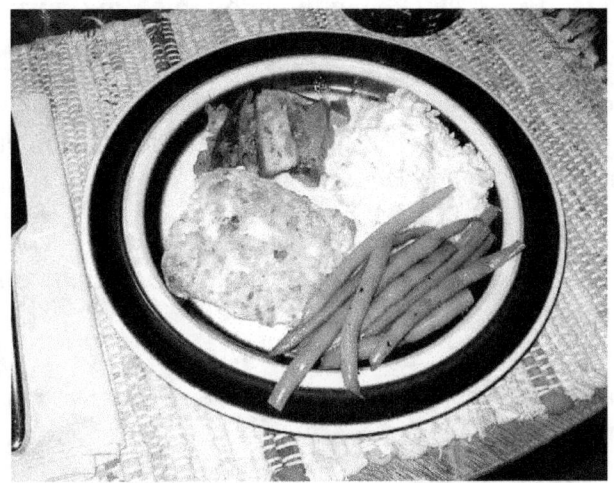

<u>Diet Tip of the Day:</u> It's worth **buying organic** for the "dirty dozen": peaches, strawberries, nectarines, apples, spinach, celery, pears, sweet bell peppers, cherries, potatoes, lettuce, and imported grapes. These fragile fruits and vegetables often require more pesticides to fight off bugs.

Day 71 - Recipe

Chicken Scaloppini

  4   skinless, boneless 6-oz chicken breast halves
  2   teaspoons fresh lemon juice
  ⅓   cup GF Panko breadcrumbs (page 215)
  ½   cup fat-free, lower-sodium GF chicken broth (page 223)
  ¼   cup dry white wine
  4   teaspoons capers
  1   tablespoon extra-virgin olive oil

Place each chicken breast half between two sheets heavy-duty plastic wrap and pound to about ¼-inch thick using meat mallet. Cut each breast in quarters. Brush chicken with lemon juice, and sprinkle with a salt and black pepper. Dredge chicken in breadcrumbs.

Heat a large nonstick skillet coated with cooking spray over medium-high heat. Add chicken to pan; cook 3 minutes on each side or until chicken is done. Remove from pan; keep warm.

Add chicken broth and white wine to pan, and cook 30 seconds, stirring constantly. Remove from heat. Stir in capers and olive oil and serve immediately.

Serves 4. 260 Calories per serving (chicken only)

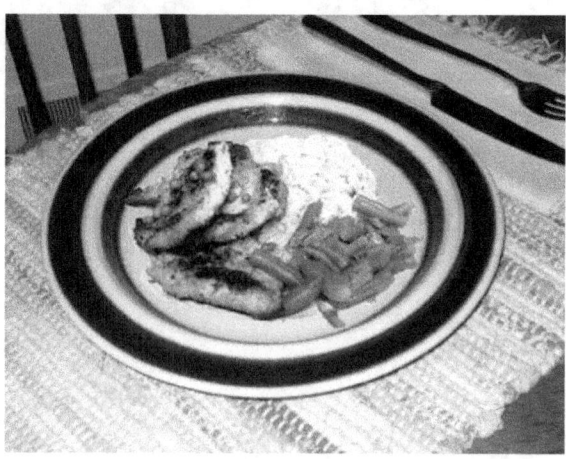

Diet Tip of the Day: Nutritionists define a "**junk food**" as a food that offers little if any essential nutrients – except calories – and often it replaces more important foods.

Day 72 - Recipe

Fish Dinner - Out

No recipe today. No cooking today. Have a fish dinner at a restaurant, but make sure you choose a restaurant where you have a good chance to eat gluten free and achieve your calorie goal. For today, your **goal for dinner is a maximum of 595 Calories**. This includes appetizer, soup, main course and dessert.

Tips for Eating Fish Out: The following is almost an exact repeat of the advice given eating out on previous days. First make sure you choose a restaurant where gluten-free food is available and where you have a good chance to achieve your calorie goal. Before you out go read the menu online and reduce your food choices so you can have more focused questions for the staff. You are more likely to get a safe meal if you call the restaurant before you go to let them know of your gluten-free needs. And call during a slow time so you can have the host's complete attention.

In the restaurant, to ensure you are served a gluten-free meal, it is important to communicate your need to eat 100 percent gluten-free assertively but pleasantly. Try to speak directly to the chef or manager. Otherwise, ask your server what is in the food and how it is prepared. Menu descriptions do not always list every ingredient. Inquire how gluten-free grains such as rice and risottos are cooked. Sometimes they are cooked in broth which may contain gluten. Confirm that separate, clean utensils and equipment will be used to prepare your meal.

Order simple, such as broiled fish with steamed vegetables and brown rice. Tell the waiter you want no sauce, no gravy, nothing added. Then, knowing your calorie objective, and that fish is about 50 Calories per ounce, most steamed vegetable servings average approximately 50 Calories per cup, and rice is about 100 Calories per ½ cup, decide how much to eat – and take the remainder home. And consider bringing your own gluten-free salad dressing to the restaurant. If fresh fruit is not an option, pass on dessert and have the evening snack specified in the *90-Day Gluten-Free Smart Diet* meal plan for that day.

In a restaurant, most nutritionists recommend you eat the low-calorie items on your plate first. Start with the salad, soup and veggies. By the time you get to the chicken and starches you will hopefully be full enough to be content with smaller portions of the higher-calorie choices.

Pasta Pomodoro

Pasta Pomodoro (Italian for pasta with tomatoes) is typically prepared with angel hair pasta, olive oil, fresh tomatoes, and fresh basil. It's light, delicious and easy to make.

¾ pound angel hair GF pasta
1½ pints cherry tomatoes (about 45), halved
8 fresh basil leaves, chopped
4 cloves garlic, minced
2 tablespoons olive oil
4 Tbsp grated parmesan cheese

Cook angel hair pasta per package directions. Over medium heat, sauté the garlic in olive oil until it just starts to turn golden. Add tomatoes and cook for about 10 minutes, or until they just start to release juices. Turn off the heat and stir basil into the sauce. Over the cooked pasta, spoon the tomato sauce with a little of the pasta water and garnish with more basil and grated cheese.

Serves 4. 420 Calories per serving

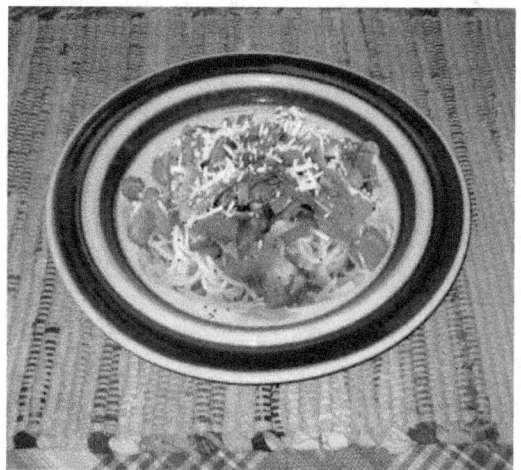

Above prepared with mix of cherry and plum tomatoes.

Diet Tip of the Day: Thinking about using **honey** rather than sugar? Honey has about 21 calories per teaspoon while sugar has 15. And the vitamin and mineral content of honey is very low.

Day 74 - Recipe

Frozen Dinner

No recipe today. No cooking today. Instead select a frozen dinner from the following:

- Amy's Quinoa, Black Beans, Butternut Squash & Chard (**240 Cal**)
- Amy's Black Bean & Cheese Enchilada (**240 Cal**)
- Amy's Mushroom Risotto Bowl (**240 Cal**)
- Amy's Sweet & Sour Asian Noodle Bowl (**250 Cal**)
- Amy's Vegetable Parmesan Bowl (**260 Cal**)
- Amy's Brown Rice & Veggies Bowl – Light in Sodium (**260 Cal**)
- Amy's Brown Rice, Black-eyed Peas & Veggies Bowl (**290 Cal**)
- Amy's Teriyaki Bowl (**290 Cal**)
- Amy's Asian Noodle Stir Fry (**300 Cal**)
- Amy's Vegetable Lasagna (**300 Cal**)
- Amy's Thai Stir-Fry (**310 Cal**)
- Amy's Tofu Scramble (**320 Cal**)

- Artisan Bistro Wild Alaskan Salmon (**200 Cal**)
- Artisan Bistro Chicken Parmesan Bake (**200 Cal**)
- Artisan Bistro Turkey Cheddar Bake (**240 Cal**)
- Artisan Bistro Wild Alaskan Salmon Bake (**240 Cal**)
- Artisan Bistro Thai Style Yellow Curry with Chicken (**240 Cal**)
- Artisan Bistro Cheddar Beef Bake (**250 Cal**)
- Artisan Bistro Sesame Ginger with Salmon (**270 Cal**)
- Artisan Bistro Coconut Lemongrass with Chicken (**270 Cal**)
- Artisan Bistro Spiced Chicken Morocco (**270 Cal**)
- Artisan Bistro Albacore Tuna Bake (**280 Cal**)
- Artisan Bistro Thai Style Red Curry with Beef (**280 Cal**)
- Artisan Bistro Chicken Citron (**280 Cal**)
- Artisan Bistro Wild Alaskan Salmon with Pesto (**310 Cal**)
- Artisan Bistro Savory Turkey (**330 Cal**)
- Artisan Bistro Southwest Style Beef (**330 Cal**)
- Artisan Bistro Ginger Chicken (**350 Cal**)
- Artisan Bistro Beef with Mushroom Sauce (**350 Cal**)
- Artisan Bistro Wild Alaskan Salmon Cake (**370 Cal**)

- Smart Ones Lemon Herb Chicken Piccata (**250 Cal**)
- Smart Ones Santa Fe Style Rice & Beans (**290 Cal**)

Also note that **340 Calories are allocated for this meal**. But almost all of the above have less than 340 Calories. Use the excess calories anyway you wish. Splurge on extra dessert or save the calories for another day!

And please read the important **Frozen-Food Safety Warning** in **Appendix D** (page 226).

<u>**Diet Tip of the Day:**</u> Many health care professionals think that eating a healthy **gluten-free diet** is one of the best things you can do for your short-term and long-term health. But a gluten-free diet must be carefully planned to make sure you get the correct amount of nutrients, vitamins and minerals..

Day 75 - Recipe

Szechuan Noodles and Pork

8	ounces GF linguine pasta
1	cup GF chicken broth (page 223)
2	tablespoon soy sauce (page 217)
8	ounces ground pork (lean)
¼	teaspoon red pepper flakes
6	scallions, cut in ½-inch pieces
1	large carrot, shredded
1	tablespoon each minced garlic and ginger
1½	tablespoons creamy peanut butter (page 222)

Cook linguine per package directions. Mix broth and soy sauce in a measuring cup.

Cook ground pork and red pepper flakes in large non-stick skillet over medium-high heat for about 5 minutes. Make sure pork is browned and no longer pink. Add scallions, carrot, garlic and ginger; cook additional 3 minutes. Stir broth mixture and peanut butter into pork. Cook until peanut butter melts and is blended.

Drain linguine, add to skillet and toss to evenly coat with sauce. (Use some cooking water if needed to keep mixture creamy.) Garnish with chopped cilantro.
Serves 4. 440 Calories per serving.

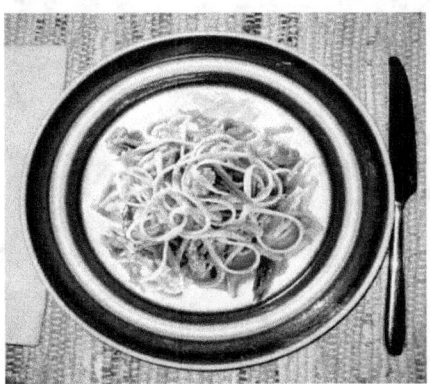

Diet Tip of the Day: Studies have shown **vegetarian** diets significantly lower the risk of colon cancer, heart disease, high blood pressure and other diseases.

Day 76 - Recipe

Gary & Sue's Grilled Scallops

We were invited by our good friends, Gary and Sue, for dinner. They prepared a simple, but nutritious low-calorie meal – which featured scallops. (Scallops are a very low calorie food – expensive but great when you're on a diet.) The photo below is our version of the main course they served that night.

1½	pounds sea scallops
3	medium tomatoes, sliced, divided
4	ears of corn
2	tablespoons olive oil, divided
1	tablespoon balsamic vinegar, divided

Place scallops in a shallow bowl. Add olive oil and vinegar and toss to coat. Grill scallops on medium-hot fire. Turn after two minutes or when first side turns opaque. Grill until second side turns opaque – about another 2 minutes. Don't overcook but test a scallop by cutting to make sure it's cooked through. Salt and black pepper to taste.

Serves 4. The food pictured on the plate below totals about 360 Calories.

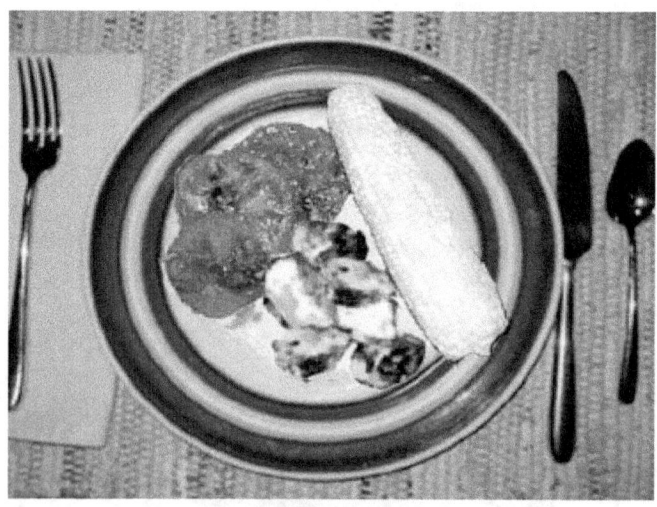

Diet Tip of the Day: When you eat fiber, it simply passes straight through, untouched by but aiding your digestive system. **Zero calories absorbed!**

Day 77 - Recipe

Chicken with Peppers and Rice

4 boneless, skinless chicken breast halves (about 1 lb)
1 red bell pepper, sliced
1 green bell pepper, sliced
1 yellow bell pepper, sliced
1 medium onion, sliced
1 teaspoon dried oregano
1 teaspoon dries basil
½ teaspoon garlic powder
2 tablespoons olive oil
¾ cup wild rice and brown rice mix

Prepare wild rice per package directions. Prepare seasoning blend of oregano, basil, garlic powder, salt and pepper. Cut chicken into 2 to 3-inch pieces. Place vegetables and chicken in re-sealable plastic bag. Add seasoning blend and olive oil. Seal bag and refrigerate for about two hours.

Preheat oven to 400°F. Place chicken and peppers in foil-lined baking pan. (Discard any remaining liquid in bag.) Bake 30 to 40 minutes, or until chicken is done. Broil an additional 2 to 3 minutes to brown chicken (optional).

Serves 4. 290 Calories per serving (Chicken, peppers and rice mix)

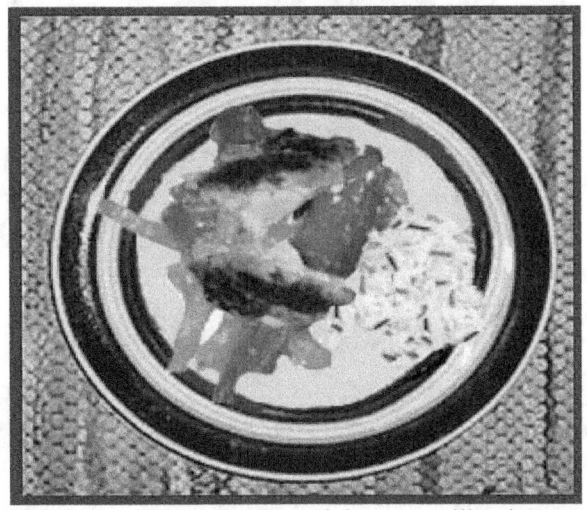

Chicken was browned too much but was still quite tasty!

Day 78 - Recipe

Trout with Lemon &Capers

4   trout fillets (4-oz each), skin attached
3   tablespoons unsalted butter, divided
2   tablespoons olive oil
2   tablespoons lemon juice
4   teaspoons chopped parsley
1   teaspoon capers
2   small lemons peeled and segmented

Score 2 crosswise slits (skin deep only) into each trout fillet using sharp knife. Turn fillets over and season flesh with the salt and pepper.

Heat 1 tablespoon butter and the olive oil in a large nonstick skillet over medium-high heat. Place the fillets in the nonstick skillet, skin side up, and cook until golden brown, about 3 minutes. Turn and continue until cooked through and the skin begins to crisp around edges, about 2 more minutes. Transfer fillets to serving dish and keep warm.

Add the remaining 2 tablespoons butter to the hot skillet and cook until just brown. Stir in the lemon juice, parsley, capers, and lemon segments. Pour sauce over fillets and serve.

Serves 4. 340 Calories per serving (trout and sauce only)

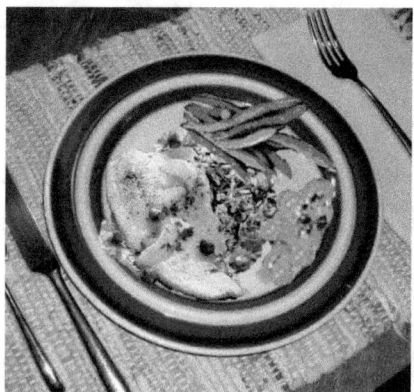

Diet Tip of the Day: Nearly every animal food, including dairy products, eggs, meat, poultry and fish are **complete proteins** because they contain all eight-essential amino acids. Soy is the only plant-based food that has all eight essential-amino acids.

Day 79 - Recipe

<u>Chinese Dinner - Out</u>

No recipe today. No cooking today. Have a Chinese dinner at your
favorite restaurant, but make sure you choose a restaurant where you
can eat gluten free and have a reasonable chance to achieve your
calorie goal. For today, **your goal for dinner is a maximum of 640
Calories**. This includes any appetizer, soup, main course and any
dessert.

Tips for Eating Chinese: Try bringing a restaurant card to the
Chinese restaurant. The cards are available online and are designed to
help explain a gluten-free diet to a waiter who might not speak English.

You can consume a lot of calories in a Chinese restaurant – if you
order carelessly. For example a typical portion of General Tso's
chicken is loaded with about 1000 Calories, then add another 200
Calories for a cup of rice.

First rule, order simple. Rice noodles prepared with vegetables or
chicken are generally a safe choice. Avoid brown sauce which may
have a soy sauce base. Instead, ask for the dish to be prepared with a
white sauce using corn starch. Then, knowing your 640 Calorie
objective, and that chicken and fish are about 50 Calories per ounce,
most steamed vegetable servings average approximately 50 Calories
per cup, and rice is about 200 Calories per cup, decide how much of the
meal you can eat – and take the remainder home. (Note that you will
be eating half a serving of left over Chinese food for lunch tomorrow.)
To stay within your maximum allowable calorie total, you should pass
on dessert and have the evening snack (if any) specified for that day in
the diet.

And although it is customary to share dishes at a Chinese
restaurant, do not permit your dinner companions to contaminate your
food. Make sure your friends do not use their gluten-contaminated
spoons to serve food from your gluten-free dish.

Incidentally, although Chinese is specified, feel free to substitute
Thai food, Vietnamese, Indian, Middle Eastern, or any other favorite
ethnic food. Just make sure you can eat gluten free and try not exceed
the maximum allowable 640 calories for this meal.

Day 80 - Recipe

<u>Vegetable Chili</u>

1 tablespoon olive oil
2 medium carrots, cut into ½-inch pieces
2 medium parsnips, cut into ½-inch pieces
1 medium onion, chopped
2 cans (15-ounces each) red kidney beans*, drained
4 teaspoons chili powder
1 can (28-ounce) whole tomatoes in juice
¼ cup fresh cilantro leaves, chopped

In saucepot, heat olive oil on medium-high. Add carrots, parsnips, chopped onion, and cook 6 to 8 minutes or until all vegetables are tender and beginning to brown, stirring occasionally.

Meanwhile, on large plate, mash 1 cup drained beans. Stir chili powder into vegetables in saucepot; cook 1 minute, stirring. Add canned tomatoes with their juice, whole and mashed beans, and 2 cups water. Heat to boiling on high, breaking up tomatoes with spoon. Reduce heat to medium and cook, uncovered for 10 minutes, stirring occasionally. Finally, stir in cilantro and serve.

Serves 4. 360 Calories per serving

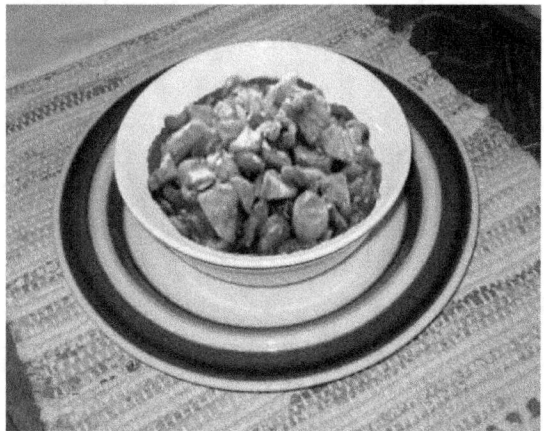

* Canned red kidney beans should be gluten free but check the ingredients on the container to be sure. Call the manufacturer and ask if the beans could contain trace gluten or could have been cross contaminated in their factory. Do not eat a food if you are not sure it is gluten free. Remember, if in doubt, go without.

Day 81 - Recipe

<u>Frozen Dinner</u>

No recipe today. No cooking today. Instead select a frozen dinner from the following:

- Amy's Quinoa, Black Beans, Butternut Squash & Chard (**240 Cal**)
- Amy's Black Bean & Cheese Enchilada (**240 Cal**)
- Amy's Mushroom Risotto Bowl (**240 Cal**)
- Amy's Sweet & Sour Asian Noodle Bowl (**250 Cal**)
- Amy's Vegetable Parmesan Bowl (**260 Cal**)
- Amy's Brown Rice & Veggies Bowl – Light in Sodium (**260 Cal**)
- Amy's Brown Rice, Black-eyed Peas & Veggies Bowl (**290 Cal**)
- Amy's Teriyaki Bowl (**290 Cal**)
- Amy's Asian Noodle Stir Fry (**300 Cal**)
- Amy's Vegetable Lasagna (**300 Cal**)
- Amy's Thai Stir-Fry (**310 Cal**)
- Amy's Tofu Scramble (**320 Cal**)

- Artisan Bistro Wild Alaskan Salmon (**200 Cal**)
- Artisan Bistro Chicken Parmesan Bake (**200 Cal**)
- Artisan Bistro Turkey Cheddar Bake (**240 Cal**)
- Artisan Bistro Wild Alaskan Salmon Bake (**240 Cal**)
- Artisan Bistro Thai Style Yellow Curry with Chicken (**240 Cal**)
- Artisan Bistro Cheddar Beef Bake (**250 Cal**)
- Artisan Bistro Sesame Ginger with Salmon (**270 Cal**)
- Artisan Bistro Coconut Lemongrass with Chicken (**270 Cal**)
- Artisan Bistro Spiced Chicken Morocco (**270 Cal**)
- Artisan Bistro Albacore Tuna Bake (**280 Cal**)
- Artisan Bistro Thai Style Red Curry with Beef (**280 Cal**)
- Artisan Bistro Chicken Citron (**280 Cal**)
- Artisan Bistro Wild Alaskan Salmon with Pesto (**310 Cal**)
- Artisan Bistro Savory Turkey (**330 Cal**)
- Artisan Bistro Southwest Style Beef (**330 Cal**)
- Artisan Bistro Ginger Chicken (**350 Cal**)
- Artisan Bistro Beef with Mushroom Sauce (**350 Cal**)
- Artisan Bistro Wild Alaskan Salmon Cake (**370 Cal**)

- Smart Ones Lemon Herb Chicken Piccata (**250 Cal**)
- Smart Ones Santa Fe Style Rice & Beans (**290 Cal**)

Also note that **340 Calories are allocated for this meal**. But almost all of the above have less than 340 Calories. Use the excess calories anyway you wish. Splurge on extra dessert or save the calories for another day!

And please read the important **Frozen-Food Safety Warning** in **Appendix D** (page 226).

<u>**Diet Tip of the Day:**</u> Keep low-calorie **lean sandwich fixings on hand** (whole-wheat bread, sliced turkey, reduced-fat cheese, lettuce, tomatoes and mustard).

Day 82 - Recipe

<u>Chinese Chicken Salad</u>

    4 skinless, boneless chicken breast halves (½ lb total)
    1 cup carrots, sliced
    1 cup red bell peppers, sliced
    4 green onions, diced
    1 cup edamame beans*, cooked and shelled
    1 cup GF chow mein noodles (page 216)
    2 hearts romaine lettuce
    4 cups mesclun mix or spring mix

<u>Chinese salad dressing</u>: In a jar with a tight-fitting lid combine 2 tsp garlic powder, 1 tsp dried parsley, 1 tsp dried basil, 1 tsp honey, 2 tsp GF soy sauce, 4 tsp sesame oil, 2 tsp Sriracha** (Chinese hot sauce – optional), 4 tsp Dijon mustard, 4 tbsp olive oil, 4 tbsp rice wine vinegar and a dash of black pepper. Shake well and set aside.

Grill chicken breast halves and then cut them into small pieces.

In a bowl, combine romaine lettuce, mesclun mix lettuces (or spring mix), carrots, red bell pepper, green onions and edamame. Add the dressing and toss. Add chow mien noodles and chicken and toss again. **<u>Serves 4</u>**. 440 Calories per serving

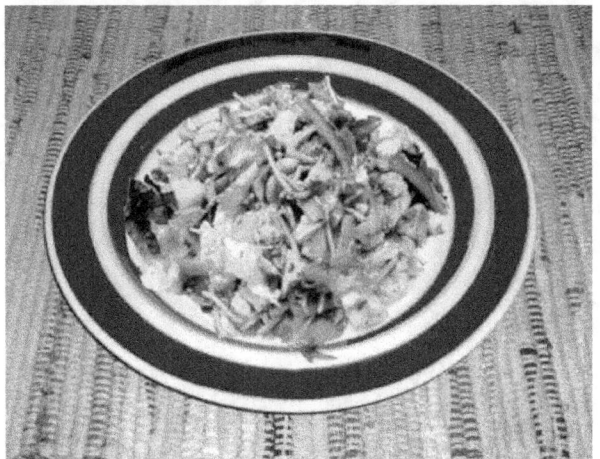

* Edamame beans are naturally gluten free. But make sure there are no added gluten-containing ingredients. ** Sriracha, is a GF Chinese hot sauce produced by Huy Fong Inc.

Day 83 - Recipe

Hearty Lentil Stew

½ cup chopped onion
2   garlic cloves, minced
1   tablespoon vegetable oil
1   cup lentils, rinsed
4   tsp GF vegetable or chicken bouillon (page 223) granules
3   tsp GF Worcestershire sauce (page 218)
1   bay leaf
1   cup chopped carrots
14.5-ounce can diced tomatoes with liquid
10-oz package frozen chopped spinach, thawed
1   Tbsp red wine vinegar

In a large saucepan, sauté onion and garlic in oil until tender. Add 5 cups of water, lentils, bouillon, Worcestershire sauce, ½ teaspoon salt, ¼ teaspoon black pepper and the bay leaf. Bring to a boil. Reduce heat; cover and simmer for 20 minutes.

Add the carrots, tomatoes and spinach; return to a boil. Reduce heat; cover and simmer additional 15 to 20 minutes, or until lentils ender. Stir in vinegar and serve.
Serves 4. 260 Calories per serving

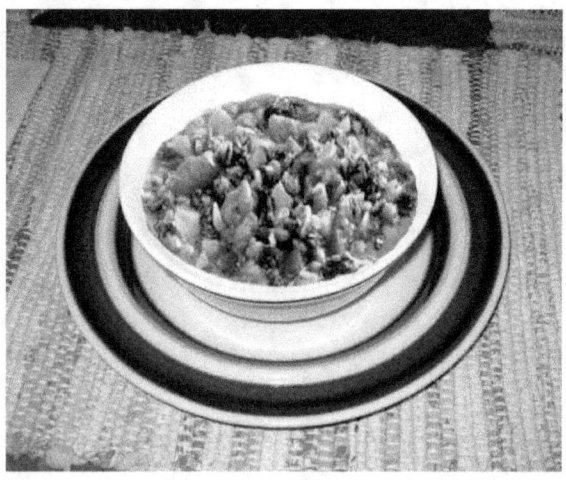

Day 84 - Recipe

<u>Turkey Burger</u>

  1¼ pounds ground turkey
  1   tablespoon GF Worcestershire sauce
  1   tablespoon GF mustard (page 217)
  1   tablespoon olive oil for brushing
  4   GF hamburger rolls (page 216)

Lightly mix together the ground turkey, Worcestershire sauce, mustard, salt and black pepper. Form into 4 patties and brush each side lightly with olive oil.

Heat grill to medium-high. Place patties on grill and cook for 3 to 4 minutes each side for medium-well done. Salt and pepper to taste. <u>**Serves 4**</u>. 355 Calories per serving (turkey burger only)

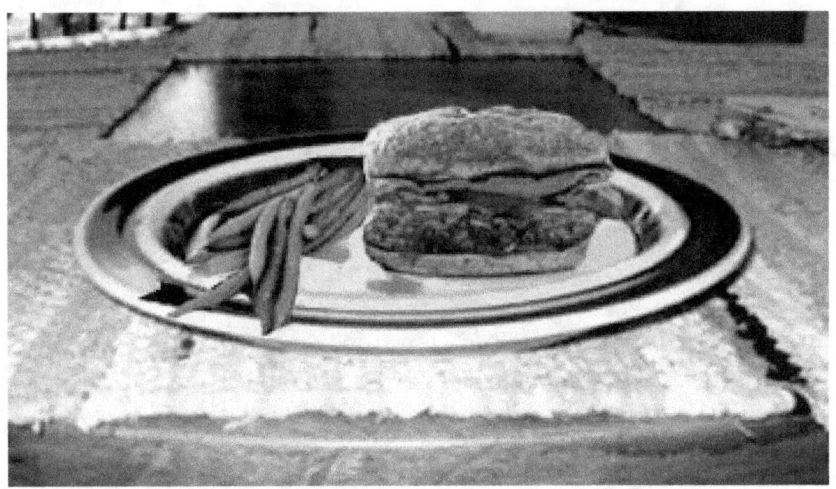

<u>**Diet Tip of the Day:**</u> Consistently **choose healthy foods**, avoid harmful foods and large portions and exercise regularly. Nothing else will control your weight over the long haul.

Carrie's Low-Cal Meat Loaf

½ pound ground white meat turkey
½ pound ground beef (about 90% lean)
1 large egg
½ cup skim milk
¼ cup GF Panko bread crumbs (page 216)
¼ cup ketchup
¼ cup chopped carrots
¼ cup chopped onion

In a medium bowl, combine all ingredients. Add salt and pepper to taste. Mix until blended and form into a loaf. Place loaf into oven preheated to 350 °F. Bake until an instant-read thermometer inserted in the center of the loaf reads 160 °F. This should take about one hour.

Shown below is meat loaf, acorn squash (baked with 1 teaspoon of maple syrup). Also shown is steamed spinach drizzled with extra-virgin olive oil. **Serves 5**. About 290 Calories per serving (for meat loaf only). Note that half a serving of left over meat loaf is to be eaten for lunch on Day 87.

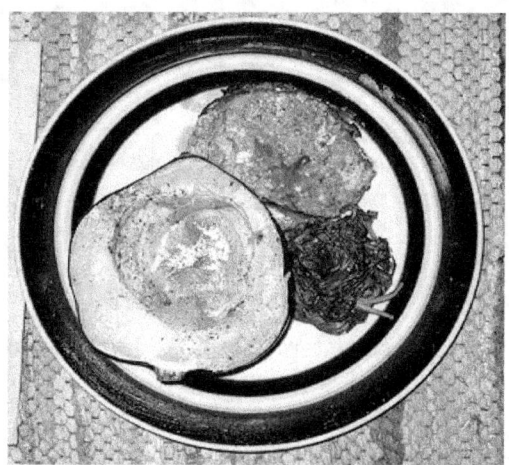

Diet Tip of the Day: Your **body weight fluctuates** two to three pounds daily. Your body weight is lowest before breakfast and highest in the evening before you retire.

Day 86 - Recipe

Tuna & Bean Salad

1	tuna steak, about 2 inches thick (14 ounces)
2	tablespoons extra-virgin olive oil
1	tablespoon lemon juice
1	garlic clove, crushed
1	tablespoon **Dijon mustard** (page 217)
1	15-ounce can cannellini beans*, drained
1	small red onion, thinly sliced
2	red peppers, seeded and thinly sliced
½	cucumber, halved lengthwise and thinly sliced
6	cups watercress

Heat a ridged grill pan coated with cooking spray over medium-high heat. Season tuna steak on both sides with coarsely ground black pepper. Cook the tuna 4 minutes on each side - the outside should be browned and the center light pink. Be careful not to overcook. Remove from the pan and set aside.

Mix together the oil, lemon juice, garlic, and mustard in a salad bowl. Season with salt and pepper to taste. Add the cannellini beans, onion, peppers, cucumber and watercress. Toss gently to mix. Cut tuna into ½-inch thick slices. Arrange on top of salad and serve with lemon wedges. **Serves 4**. 355 Calories per serving

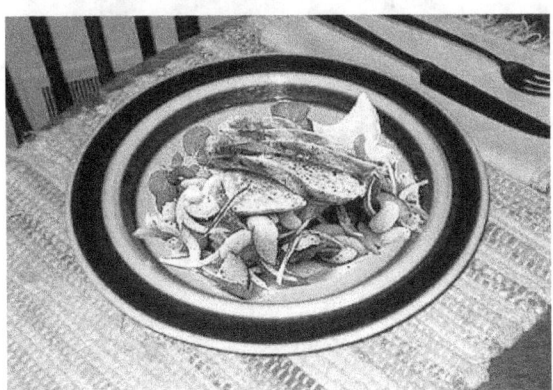

* Canned cannellini beans should be gluten free but check the ingredients on the container to be sure. Call the manufacturer and ask if the beans could contain trace gluten or could have been cross contaminated in their factory. Do not eat a food if you are not sure it is gluten free. Remember, if in doubt, go without.

Day 87 - Recipe

<u>Pasta Primavera</u>

¾ pound GF penne pasta (page 222)
2 cups broccoli florets
1 red bell pepper, sliced
1 carrot, cut to 1-inch sticks
½ cup frozen green peas & ½ cup frozen sweet corn
1 small onion, chopped
1 tablespoon minced garlic
3 tablespoons olive oil
1 teaspoon fresh basil, chopped

Cook penne pasta per package directions. Drain and place pasta in a bowl. Pre-cook the carrot and broccoli florets.

In a large heavy skillet, heat the olive oil and sauté onion and garlic until lightly golden. Add vegetables and sauté until the peppers are soft. Combine sautéed vegetables in the bowl with the pasta. Toss well. Garnish with chopped basil, season to taste, and top with freshly grated Parmesan cheese.

<u>**Serves 4**</u>. 460 Calories per serving

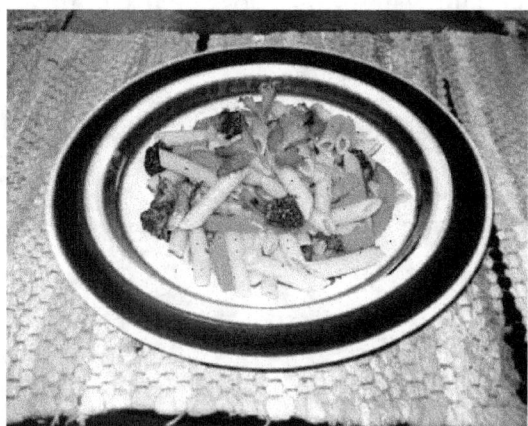

Photo taken before grated cheese was added.

<u>**Diet Tip of the Day**</u>: When possible, **select fresh and natural foods** and whole-grain products. Avoid chemical preservatives and additives, artificial and imitation foods, refined and processed foods, and foods that are comprised of "nutritionally-empty calories."

Day 88 - Recipe

Frozen Dinner

No recipe today. No cooking today. Instead select a frozen dinner from the following:

- Amy's Quinoa, Black Beans, Butternut Squash & Chard (**240 Cal**)
- Amy's Black Bean & Cheese Enchilada (**240 Cal**)
- Amy's Mushroom Risotto Bowl (**240 Cal**)
- Amy's Sweet & Sour Asian Noodle Bowl (**250 Cal**)
- Amy's Vegetable Parmesan Bowl (**260 Cal**)
- Amy's Brown Rice & Veggies Bowl – Light in Sodium (**260 Cal**)
- Amy's Brown Rice, Black-eyed Peas & Veggies Bowl (**290 Cal**)
- Amy's Teriyaki Bowl (**290 Cal**)
- Amy's Asian Noodle Stir Fry (**300 Cal**)
- Amy's Vegetable Lasagna (**300 Cal**)
- Amy's Thai Stir-Fry (**310 Cal**)
- Amy's Tofu Scramble (**320 Cal**)

- Artisan Bistro Wild Alaskan Salmon (**200 Cal**)
- Artisan Bistro Chicken Parmesan Bake (**200 Cal**)
- Artisan Bistro Turkey Cheddar Bake (**240 Cal**)
- Artisan Bistro Wild Alaskan Salmon Bake (**240 Cal**)
- Artisan Bistro Thai Style Yellow Curry with Chicken (**240 Cal**)
- Artisan Bistro Cheddar Beef Bake (**250 Cal**)
- Artisan Bistro Sesame Ginger with Salmon (**270 Cal**)
- Artisan Bistro Coconut Lemongrass with Chicken (**270 Cal**)
- Artisan Bistro Spiced Chicken Morocco (**270 Cal**)
- Artisan Bistro Albacore Tuna Bake (**280 Cal**)
- Artisan Bistro Thai Style Red Curry with Beef (**280 Cal**)
- Artisan Bistro Chicken Citron (**280 Cal**)
- Artisan Bistro Wild Alaskan Salmon with Pesto (**310 Cal**)
- Artisan Bistro Savory Turkey (**330 Cal**)
- Artisan Bistro Southwest Style Beef (**330 Cal**)
- Artisan Bistro Ginger Chicken (**350 Cal**)
- Artisan Bistro Beef with Mushroom Sauce (**350 Cal**)
- Artisan Bistro Wild Alaskan Salmon Cake (**370 Cal**)

- Smart Ones Lemon Herb Chicken Piccata (**250 Cal**)
- Smart Ones Santa Fe Style Rice & Beans (**290 Cal**)

Also note that **340 Calories are allocated for this meal**. But almost all of the above have less than 340 Calories. Use the excess calories anyway you wish. Splurge on extra dessert or save the calories for another day!

Please read the important **Frozen-Food Safety Warning** in **Appendix D** (page 226).

<u>**Diet Tip of the Day:**</u> Understand that the only **sure way to slim down for keeps** is to eat less and exercise more. There are no safe short cuts or miracle methods for taking off weight.

Day 89 - Recipe

Fish Stew

1	pound shrimp, peeled and de-veined
¾	pound skinless flounder fillet, cut into strips
1	pound new baby potatoes, halved
2	peppers (red and yellow) sliced into strips
1	onion, halved and sliced
4	ounces white wine
2	cups GF vegetable stock (page 223)
2	cloves garlic, crushed
1	small bunch basil, shredded
1½	tablespoons olive oil

In a large pot, sauté garlic, onion and peppers in olive oil until they are completely softened. Stir in wine, vegetable stock and potatoes. Simmer until potatoes are tender.

Add the shrimp and flounder and cook for additional 4 minutes. Stir in basil and serve.

Serves 4. 300 Calories per serving

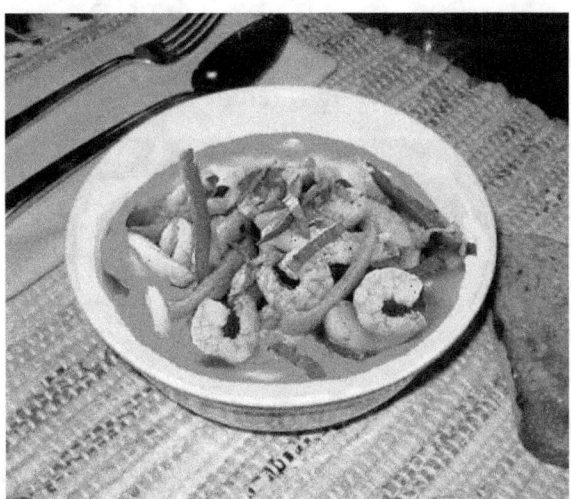

Diet Tip of the Day: All **fish** are relatively low-calorie foods and are good sources of protein and fat-soluble vitamins A and D.

Day 90 - Recipe

<u>Veal with Mushrooms & Tomato</u>

½ pound GF spaghetti
¾ pound veal cutlets
8 ounces sliced mushrooms
2 tablespoon olive oil, divided
2 tablespoons all purpose GF flour
3 green onions, small, sliced
½ cup GF chicken broth (page 223)
14.5-ounce can diced tomatoes

Pound veal to about ¼-inch thickness. Rinse, pat dry and cut into 2-inch pieces. Heat 1 tablespoon olive oil in large nonstick skillet over medium heat. Add mushrooms and cook, stirring, until lightly browned. Remove and set aside.

Season veal with salt and pepper and coat lightly with flour. Add remaining olive oil to skillet and cook veal over medium heat for about 2 minutes on each side, or until browned. Add the green onions and cook for 1 minute longer. Add chicken broth and cook, uncovered, for 5 minutes. Add tomatoes; cover and simmer for 3 to 5 minutes. Serve over spaghetti cooked per package directions.

<u>Serves 4</u>. 520 Calories per serving (includes spaghetti)

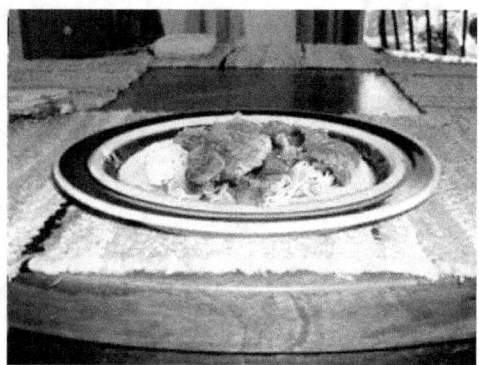

<u>Diet Tip of the Day:</u> Successful weight loss and subsequent weight maintenance **requires knowledge, desire and discipline**. Avoid the latest fad diets. Instead, take the time to develop a true understanding of weight control and then change your eating and activity habits accordingly.

Appendix A
Gluten Notes

Celiac Disease: The primary reason for a gluten-free diet is to combat celiac disease which is a chronic, systemic, autoimmune disorder that causes intestinal damage. Common celiac symptoms include diarrhea, abdominal pain, weight loss and fatigue. On the other hand, some celiac suffers experience constipation instead of diarrhea, weight gain instead of weight loss and heartburn instead of stomach pain. And a few people diagnosed with celiac disease have almost no symptoms. In net, celiac affects many body systems in different ways and because every person displays celiac disease differently, it is a difficult condition to diagnose. A strict gluten-free diet most often alleviates celiac-related symptoms. Keep in mind that all of these possible celiac disease symptoms can be caused by other medical problems. If you suspect you have celiac disease, make sure to see a physician.

Non Celiac Gluten Sensitivity: Another reason to go gluten free is to combat a condition called non-celiac gluten sensitivity that can also affect nearly every system in the body with symptoms that include digestive complaints, skin problems, brain fog, joint pain and numbness in extremities. Because research into this condition is in its early stages, not all physicians have accepted it as an illness and as a result not all physicians provide patients with a diagnosis of gluten sensitivity. Nevertheless, if you believe you suffer from gluten sensitivity, see a physician. To make matters even more confusing, some people are allergic to wheat. These people experience typical allergy symptoms (nasal congestion, etc) and sometimes they also have gastrointestinal symptoms.

Healthier Way to Lose Weight: A new reason to go gluten free is that some medical practitioners believe it is a healthier way to lose weight. But gluten-free weight loss is a recent concept and to date there has not been any research that confirms going gluten free promotes weight loss. Many physicians, however, report a considerable number of their patients claim that when they went gluten free they lost weight and felt a lot better.

Gluten Restriction Levels: Because people with celiac disease and gluten sensitivity have remarkably varying degrees of reaction to trace levels of gluten, it is useful to think in terms of three levels of gluten restriction:

The first level consists of adults with celiac disease. These individuals have a medical reason for being on a gluten-free diet and have serious reactions to gluten. They should avoid not only obvious gluten-laden foods, but also should avoid processed foods that have trace amounts of gluten as well as gluten-free foods that have been cross-contaminated by gluten foods or by trace gluten. (The obvious gluten-laden foods include bread, cereals, and all products with wheat, barley or rye as an ingredient.)

The second level of gluten restriction consists of individuals with non-celiac gluten sensitivity or a wheat allergy who may or may not have a reaction to trace gluten in their food. These people should avoid the obvious gluten containing foods and by trial and error learn what supposedly gluten-free foods (that nevertheless might contain trace gluten) they should also avoid.

In the third level are those who only want to lose weight and feel better on a gluten free diet. These people have only to avoid obvious gluten-containing foods.

Eating Gluten Free in Brief: First, you should be aware of food label ingredients that mean that gluten grains are present: these are triticum vulgare (wheat), triticum spelta (a form of wheat), triticale (cross between wheat and rye), hordeum vulgare (barley) and secale cereale (rye).

Any of the following ingredients on a label indicate that the food definitely contains gluten: wheat protein, hydrolyzed wheat protein, wheat starch, hydrolyzed wheat starch, wheat flour, bread flour, bleached flour, bulgur (a form of wheat), malt (made from barley), couscous (made from wheat), farina (made from wheat), pasta (made from wheat unless otherwise indicated), seitan (made from wheat gluten and commonly found in vegetarian meals) and wheat germ oil or extract (likely cross contaminated).

Any of the following on a label indicate that the food might contain gluten: vegetable protein, hydrolyzed vegetable protein (could be from wheat, corn or soy), modified starch, modified food starch (can come from several sources, including wheat), natural flavor (can be made from barley), artificial flavor (can come from barley), modified food starch, hydrolyzed plant protein (HPP), hydrolyzed vegetable protein (HVP), seasonings, flavorings, vegetable starch, dextrin (sometimes made from wheat) and maltodextrin (sometimes made from wheat).

If a product contains wheat, the FDA requires that it be stated on the food's label. But other gluten-containing grains (barley or rye) do not have to be declared although they might have been added to a food's ingredients. If in doubt, check with the food manufacturer to determine if a food is truly gluten free. (Incidentally, when you call a manufacturer, it is not unusual for them to offer discount coupons for their products!)

Gluten Cross Contamination: Of course, a food that has no gluten-containing ingredients could be cross contaminated with gluten. For example, soybeans and oats do not naturally contain gluten. But soybeans and oats are frequently grown in rotation with wheat crops. That means farmers often use the same fields to grow soy, oats and wheat, they use the same combines to harvest the crops, the same storage facilities and the same trucks to transport the crops to market. As a result, soy and oats are often gluten cross-contaminated.

So if you react to a food that is not supposed to have any gluten ingredients, it is probably because the food contains trace gluten due to cross contamination. The food might have just enough trace gluten to give you problems, despite having an apparently safe list of ingredients.

Appreciate that reactions to gluten vary from person to person. And a gluten reaction is influenced not only by how much gluten is in a food, but also by how much of that food you eat.

Gluten-Free Labeling Standards: The quantity of gluten in a particular product is expressed as parts of gluten contained in a million parts of the product, stated as parts per million, or ppm of gluten. In 2013, the U.S. Food and Drug Administration allowed food manufacturers to label products "gluten-free" that contain less than 20 ppm of gluten (GF 20). Canada the UK and most European Union countries also consider 20 ppm to be gluten free. (20 ppm means a product contains 0.002% gluten). Some people, however, still react to products labeled "gluten-free" that contain less than 20 ppm of gluten. Because of this, several food manufacturers maintain more rigorous standards, typically lowering the amount of gluten in a product to less than 5 or 10 ppm.

Appendix B
Gluten-Free Foods

Because food ingredients and formulations can change at any time, the following lists and recommendations should only be used as a guide. Read the food label and ingredient statement on the food package carefully at the time of purchase to ensure it is gluten free. Moreover, recall that only people with celiac disease and those with extreme gluten sensitivity usually need to be concerned with trace gluten.

And keep in mind our gluten-free guideline: "If in doubt, go without." Do not eat a supposedly gluten-free food if there is no ingredient list or if you are not sure whether the ingredients are gluten-free. If you are unsure of the ingredients, call the food manufacturer for more information.

Finally, although the following list is reasonably comprehensive, it does not contain all the gluten-free foods being sold. And more gluten-free products are continually being developed and found on store shelves.

Baking Mixes, etc: Any baking mix you buy should be labeled "gluten-free." Most baking supplies, such as baking soda, sugar and cocoa, are considered gluten-free, but check ingredients to make certain. Davis, Rumford, Bob's Red Mill and Clabber Girl's baking powder are gluten free.

All Purpose Flour: Bob's Red Mill, King Arthur and other mills make gluten-free all-purpose flour.

Corn Meal: Corn meal should be safe but check the label carefully. Bob's Red Mill makes corn meal in gluten-free factory.

Pancake Mix: Bob's Red Mill, King Arthur, Bisquick and others make gluten free pancake mix.

Pizza Dough: Bob's Red Mill and King Arthur also make gluten free pizza dough.

Bread Products: The gluten in wheat, barley and rye consists of two proteins that combine during the baking process to form a substance that provides bread and other baked goods with elasticity and structure. Gluten also helps bread dough rise into a light, airy loaf. Other grains do not have these characteristics, which is why it is difficult to find passable gluten-free bread. These days many supermarkets stock gluten-free bread, but you often can find a better selection online.

Bread: Udi's Whole Grain Bread (65 Calories per slice), Udi's White Sandwich Bread (70 Calories per slice) and Udi's Cinnamon Raisin Bread (70 Calories per slice), as well as many others are gluten free.

Bread Crumbs: Kinnikinnick Panko-Style Bread Crumbs are gluten free.

Chow Mein Noodles: Goldberg's makes GF chow mein noodles. They are sold in Walmart and many supermarkets.

Hamburger Buns: Kinnikinnick's Hamburger Buns (150 Calories), Rudi's Multi-Grain Hamburger Buns (190 Calories) and Udi's Classic and Whole-Grain Hamburger Buns (190 and 180 Calories per bun) are all gluten free.

Hot Dog Buns: Kinnikinnick's Hot Dog Buns (150 Calories), Rudi's Multi-Grain Hot Dog Buns (140 Calories) and Udi's Classic and Whole-Grain Hot Dog Buns (190 Calories) are all gluten free.

Pita Bread: Toufayan (110 Calories) sells gluten-free wraps.

Polenta: Bob's Red Mill Gluten Free Corn Grits/Polenta is gluten free.

Cereals: Some major brands now make several gluten-free cereals:
- General Mills Rice Chex (100 Calories per cup)
- General Mills Corn Chex (120 Calories per cup)
- General Mills Vanilla Chex (120 Calories per ¾ cup)
- General Mills Cinnamon Chex (120 Calories per ¾ cup)
- General Mills Chocolate Chex (130 Calories per ¾ cup)
- General Mills Apple Cinnamon Chex (130 Calories per ¾ cup)
- General Mills Honey Nut Chex (120 Calories per ¾ cup)
- Glutino Honey Nut (120 Calories per ¾ cup)
- Glutino Apple Cinnamon (120 Calories per ¾ cup).
- Kellogg's Rice Krispies - gluten-free (110 Calories per cup)
- Cream of Rice (150 Calories per packet)
- Bob's Red Mill Oat Meal
- GF Harvest Oat Meal (150 Calories per ½ cup)
- Waffles: Van's makes six varieties of gluten free waffles.

Coffee, Tea, Soda, Fruit Drinks and Alcohol: Unflavored coffee and black or green tea should be gluten-free, but flavored varieties may not be. Most popular sodas in the United States are gluten-free. Juice that is 100 percent fruit should be gluten-free, but fruit drinks made from fruit plus other ingredients may not be. Conventional beer contains gluten; whereas, wine is gluten-free.

Condiments, Spices & Sauces: In most cases, you will need to check ingredients or call the manufacturer to determine whether their product is gluten free.

BBQ sauces: Sweet Baby Ray's BBQ Sauce (35 Calories per tablespoon any variety), and KC Masterpiece BBQ Sauce (30 Calories per tablespoon any variety) are gluten free.

Cajun Herb-Spice Mix: Cajun's Choice Blackened and Creole Seasoning, Cajun Quick Shake Seasonings and McCormick's Cajun Seasoning are gluten free.

Herb's & Spices: . Regular salt and pepper should be gluten-free. Fresh herbs and spices in a store's produce section are safe. McCormick's single ingredient spices are gluten-free to 20 parts per million and their spice blends like Italian Seasoning and Salad Supreme Seasoning are gluten free. Check other spice manufacturers for possible gluten cross-contamination.

Marinades: Bone Suckin' Original (also Poultry, Seafood & Steak) Seasoning & Rub and Kikkoman Gluten-Free Teriyaki Marinade & Sauce.

Mustard & Ketchup: French's yellow mustard and Heinz ketchup are gluten-free.

Salsas: The following salsas are gluten free to 20 ppm. All varieties have 5 to 8 Calories per tablespoon.
- Amy's Salsa (mild & medium)
- Amy's Black Bean & Corn
- Farmer's Garden Salsa (medium & hot)
- Farmer's Peach
- Farmer's Pineapple
- Farmer's Roasted Garlic
- Newman's Own Black Bean & Corn
- Ortega Black Bean & Corn
- Ortega Garden Vegetable
- Ortega Original
- Ortega Thick & Chunky
- Ortega Salsa Verde

Soy Sauce: San-J and Kikkoman make gluten-free soy sauce.

Tomato Sauce: The following tomato sauces are both gluten free and low calorie:

- Classico Tomato & Basil Sauce (90 Calories per cup)
- Prego Light Smart Italian Sauce (90 Calories per cup)
- Hunt's Tomato Sauces (80 Calories per cup).
Tomato Paste: Hunt's is gluten free.
Canned Tomatoes: Most canned tomatoes are safe including (but not limited to) Hunt's, Del Monte and Contadina.
Vinegar: Distilled vinegar is derived from gluten grains but usually tests below the 20 ppm gluten threshold and is generally considered safe. Quite a few people with celiac and gluten sensitivity, however, report that they react to both distilled vinegar and distilled alcohol. To be safe, look for cider or balsamic vinegar rather than distilled vinegar.
Worcestershire Sauce: Lea & Perrins and French's Worcestershire Sauce are gluten free. Read the ingredients to make sure nothing has changed.

Cookies & Energy Bars: There are quite a few good tasting gluten-free cookies on the market:
- Glutino's Chocolate Chip cookies, about 60 Calories each
- Glutino's Chocolate Vanilla Creme cookies, about 60 Calories each
- Glutino's Vanilla Creme cookies, about 65 Calories each
- Kinnikinnick's Ginger Snap cookies, about 40 Calories each
- Udi's Chocolate Chip cookies, about 95 Calories each
- Udi's Ginger cookies, about 90 Calories each
- Udi's Oatmeal Raisin cookies, about 90 Calories each
- Udi's Snicker Doodle cookies, about 90 Calories each
Energy Bars: An energy bar is a convenient and sometimes healthy snack. But be careful to choose a brand that comes with protein, vitamins, and minerals, rather than high fructose, corn syrup or sugar. The following are five gluten-free energy bar manufacturers. (There are others.)
- Bumble Bar Organic Energy Bar (about 200 Calories per bar)
- Macrobars Organic Peanut Protein (about 260 Calories)
- NuGo 10 Raw Natural Energy Bar (200 Calories)
- Pure Organic Raw Fruit & Nut Bar (about 200 Calories)
- Raw Revolution Organic Food Bar (about 230 Calories).

Frozen Entrees: Most larger supermarkets have a reasonably good selection of frozen entrees. At this writing, Amy's and Artisan Bistro sell more gluten-free frozen entrees than any other manufacturer. Smart Ones makes two gluten-free entrees. Glutino offers two gluten-free frozen entrees but each contain 400 Calories and are not in the following list:

- Amy's Quinoa, Black Beans, Butternut Squash & Chard (**240 Cal**)
- Amy's Black Bean & Cheese Enchilada (**240 Cal**)
- Amy's Mushroom Risotto Bowl (**240 Cal**)
- Amy's Sweet & Sour Asian Noodle Bowl (**250 Cal**)
- Amy's Vegetable Parmesan Bowl (**260 Cal**)
- Amy's Brown Rice & Veggies Bowl – Light in Sodium (**260 Cal**)
- Amy's Brown Rice, Black-eyed Peas & Veggies Bowl (**290 Cal**)
- Amy's Teriyaki Bowl (**290 Cal**)
- Amy's Asian Noodle Stir Fry (**300 Cal**)
- Amy's Vegetable Lasagna (**300 Cal**)
- Amy's Thai Stir-Fry (**310 Cal**)
- Amy's Tofu Scramble (**320 Cal**)

- Artisan Bistro Wild Alaskan Salmon (**200 Cal**)
- Artisan Bistro Chicken Parmesan Bake (**200 Cal**)
- Artisan Bistro Turkey Cheddar Bake (**240 Cal**)
- Artisan Bistro Wild Alaskan Salmon Bake (**240 Cal**)
- Artisan Bistro Thai Style Yellow Curry with Chicken (**240 Cal**)
- Artisan Bistro Cheddar Beef Bake (**250 Cal**)
- Artisan Bistro Sesame Ginger with Salmon (**270 Cal**)
- Artisan Bistro Coconut Lemongrass with Chicken (**270 Cal**)
- Artisan Bistro Spiced Chicken Morocco (**270 Cal**)
- Artisan Bistro Albacore Tuna Bake (**280 Cal**)
- Artisan Bistro Thai Style Red Curry with Beef (**280 Cal**)
- Artisan Bistro Chicken Citron (**280 Cal**)
- Artisan Bistro Wild Alaskan Salmon with Pesto (**310 Cal**)
- Artisan Bistro Savory Turkey (**330 Cal**)
- Artisan Bistro Southwest Style Beef (**330 Cal**)
- Artisan Bistro Ginger Chicken (**350 Cal**)
- Artisan Bistro Beef with Mushroom Sauce (**350 Cal**)
- Artisan Bistro Wild Alaskan Salmon Cake (**370 Cal**)

- Smart Ones Lemon Herb Chicken Piccata (**250 Cal**)
- Smart Ones Santa Fe Style Rice & Beans (**290 Cal**)

Fruits and Vegetables: Fresh fruits, berries, greens and vegetables are naturally gluten free and generally safe. Most canned fruits and vegetables are gluten-free, but some are not. Single-ingredient frozen fruits and vegetables are generally gluten free, but frozen fruits and vegetables with multiple ingredients frequently contain gluten. Generally, more ingredients in a food increase the chance for trace gluten. Read labels carefully or contact the manufacturer to determine if a particular product is processed in a factory or on manufacturing lines shared with gluten-containing products.

Legumes and Rice: Legumes (lentils, beans, etc) are naturally gluten free, but there is always the risk of cross-contamination during processing and handling. And be wary of canned lentils, beans, etc that have added ingredients. "If in doubt, go without."

Brown Rice, white rice, long-grained rice, sticky rice and wild rice are all naturally gluten-free.

Meat, Poultry & Fish: Fresh meat, poultry and fish generally are safe on a gluten-free diet if they are not gluten cross-contaminated at a supermarket or butcher shop. (Realize that the display cases in many stores contain fans that circulate air that could cross-contaminate unprotected meat, poultry and fish. When in doubt choose meat, poultry and fish covered in plastic wrap.)

On the other hand, packaged processed meats, such as hams, bacon, sausages and luncheon meats, could contain gluten. Look for packaged processed meat products labeled gluten-free. Beware of meats and poultry with added ingredients that make them ready-to-cook meals. Most are not safe on a gluten-free diet because the store might have used unsafe ingredients when repackaging the food. Avoid these products.

There are plenty of gluten-free **deli meats**. All of Boar's Head's products are gluten-free and Hormel and Hillshire Farms both make packaged gluten-free meats. But be wary of cross-contamination by shared slicing machines at the deli counter. To make sure deli meat or cheese are gluten free, choose pre-packaged products.

There are lots of **hams** that are considered gluten-free to 20 ppm, although most are not labeled gluten-free. Again check with the manufacturer.

GF **bacon** is widely available. A partial list includes: Applegate Farms, Boar's Head, Jones Dairy Farm, and Wellshire Farms. The following is a partial list of low-calorie gluten-free bacon: Jones Turkey Bacon (35 Calories per slice) and Wellshire Farms Turkey Bacon (40 Calories per slice).

Many **hot dogs** are gluten-free, and a few are labeled gluten-free. A partial list follows: Jennie-O Turkey Franks (95 Calories each), Applegate Chicken Hot Dog (60 Calories each) and Turkey Hot Dog (50 Calories each).

The following is a partial listing of GF **burger patties**: Jennie-O Turkey Burgers (200 Calories each), Applegate Turkey Burgers (140 Calories each) and Beef Burgers (195 Calories each).

GF **veggie burgers** are produced by Amy's, Dr Praeger's and others: Amy's Bistro Veggie Burger (110 Calories) and Sonoma Veggie Burger (140 Calories) and Dr. Praeger's California Veggie Burger (110 Calories).

Many **sausages** contain bread crumbs as a filler, so check labels carefully before buying. In addition, even if the sausage does not include a gluten ingredient, it may have been manufactured on equipment that also processes gluten-containing sausage. The following is a partial list of GF sausage manufacturers: Al Fresco, Applegate Farms, Jones Dairy Farm, Smithfield and Wellshire Farms. (We just taste tested an Al Fresco chicken sausage, and found it to be tasty, low calorie and gluten-free. Al Fresco sausages are sold in many supermarkets.)

Canned **tuna and salmon** produced by Chicken of the Sea and by Bubble Bee are gluten free.

Milk and Dairy Products: Most milk and many dairy-based products are gluten-free.
 Plain, unflavored milk, butter, plain yogurt, fresh eggs and many cheeses are gluten-free. Some ice creams are gluten-free. And many flavored yogurts are gluten-free. Check the ingredients to be sure.
Milk Substitutes: Soy, rice and almond milk are most often gluten-free, but some are not. Check the labels. (Soy, rice and almond milk may be substituted for cow's skim milk provided the calorie count is close.)
Yogurt: All varieties of Chobani and Yoplait yogurt, including flavored varieties, are gluten free. At this writing, Yoplait Light in the 6 oz container has 90 Calories.
Cheeses: Most cheeses are naturally gluten-free. One slice (1 oz) of light cheese has about 70 Calories. Beware of cheese that has been sliced and repackaged at a supermarket. It might be cross contaminated. Usually, it is safer to buy cheese that has been packaged at the manufacturer's plant.
Cottage Cheese: Breakstone, Cabot, Humboldt and others make fat free, gluten-free cottage cheese.
Ice Cream: Although many ice cream products are gluten free, some are not. Also consider GF frozen fruit pops. All of Skinny Cow's ice cream

Pasta: Fortunately, there are a number of gluten-free pastas available, in different shapes and sizes. Choose gluten-free pasta made from rice or corn rather than wheat. Surprisingly, many of these gluten-free varieties are quite good, making it possible to serve gluten-free pasta whose taste is very close to wheat-based pasta. The following manufacturers make gluten-free pasta: Ancient Harvest, Andean Dream, Bionaturae, Jovial, DeBoles, DeLallo, Le Veneziane, Lundberg, Riso Bello, Rizopia, Ronzoni bars are gluten free: Chocolate Truffle Bar (100 Calories), Caramel Truffle Bar (100 Calories) and Fudge Bars (110 Calories).

Oils, Nuts & Popcorn: Most oils (olive, canola, etc), nuts, and popcorn varieties are gluten free. Nuts are naturally gluten free. But beware of nuts and popcorn with added flavorings that might contain gluten. Some popcorn brands that are considered gluten free are Jolly Time, Newman's Own and Orville Redenbacher's.
Peanut Butter: Arrowhead Mills and Smart Balance peanut butter are gluten free (about 95 Calories per tablespoon.)
Mayonnaise: Hellmann's and Best Foods regular and light mayonnaise are gluten free. (light is 35 Calories per serving)
Non-Stick Cooking Spray: Original Pam, Mazola and Wegman's store brand cooking sprays are gluten free.
Rustichella D'Abruzzo, Sam Mills and Tinkyada.

Salad Dressings: When buying vinaigrette-type salad dressings look for cider or balsamic vinegar, not distilled vinegar on the food label. (Distilled vinegar is made from gluten grains.) The following salad dressings are gluten free:
- Annie's Lite Raspberry Vinaigrette (20 Cal per tablespoon)
- Annie's Lite Italian Dressing (23 Cal per tablespoon)
- Annie's Lite Honey Mustard Vinaigrette (20 Cal per tablespoon)
- Annie's Lite Herb Balsamic Vinaigrette (25 Cal per tablespoon)
- Annie's Lite Gingerly Vinaigrette (20 Cal per tablespoon).
- Gazebo Room Lite Greek Salad Dressing (20 Cal per tablespoon)
- Ken's Lite Italian w/ Romano & Red Pepper (23 Cal per tablespoon)
- Newman's Own Lite Balsamic Vinaigrette (13 Cal per tablespoon)
- Newman's Own Lite Roasted Garlic Balsamic (25 Cal per tablespoon)

- Newman's Own Lite Red Wine Vinaigrette & Olive Oil (25 Cal per tablespoon)
- Newman's Own Lite Low-Fat Sesame Ginger (18 Calories per tablespoon)
- San-J's Tamari Sesame Salad Dressing (20 Calories per tablespoon)
- San-J's Tamari Ginger Salad Dressing (13 Calories per tablespoon)
- Sophia's Oil-Free Cilantro & Lime (5 Calories per tablespoon)

Soups **(See Appendix C for a list of GF soup.)**
Amy's Kitchen: A great many of Amy's 29 soups are considered gluten-free to 20 ppm.
Bookbinders Specialties: This gourmet soup company has 11 gluten-free soups. All are tested to below 20 ppm, and are available by mail order or in U.S. supermarkets in the northeast.
Frontier Soup: Frontier makes 28 varieties of gluten-free soup mixes. All are certified to below 5ppm of gluten. Frontier Soup mixes are available online and at upscale supermarket chains.
Imagine Foods: Imagine Foods claims all varieties of its soups are gluten-free to 20 ppm except for Organic Creamy Chicken and Imagine Bistro Bisques. Imagine soups are usually found in the "natural foods" section of supermarkets.
Pacific Foods: Almost all Pacific's soups are gluten free. Most often Pacific soups are found in the natural or health food section of a supermarket, although in some stores they are next to conventional soups.
Progresso: Choose from Progresso's many gluten-fee varieties tested to 20 ppm.
Stock, Broth & Bouillon: Stock is made by simmering vegetables, bones, meat scraps, etc, and is the best base for soups, stews, and sauces.
Unfortunately stock is rarely found on supermarket shelves. Broth is stock with added salt and can be used in the same way as homemade stock -- although broth is not as rich and complex as stock. Bouillon is dehydrated stock formed into cubes or granules. It is convenient but is typically processed with large amounts of sodium and other additives. Thus the liquid it produces is almost flavorless.

Kitchen Basics makes gluten free Chicken, Beef, Vegetable, Turkey, Seafood, Veal, Unsalted Chicken and Unsalted Beef stock. Pacific Foods sells gluten free vegetable broth, mushroom broth, beef broth and chicken and vegetable stock. College Inn's garden-

vegetable broth, organic-beef broth, tender-beef bold stock and white wine & herb broth are all
considered gluten-free to 20ppm. Hormel's vegetable, beef and chicken bouillon cubes are gluten free.

Miscellaneous
We put food products in this category that did not seem to fit anywhere else.
Pancake Syrup: Hungry Jack Lite Syrup (25 Calories per tablespoon), Log Cabin Lite Syrup (25 Calories per tablespoon) and Vermont Maid Lite Syrup (30 Calories per tablespoon) are gluten free.

Appendix C
Gluten-Free Soup

Soup Description	Calories*
Amy's Vegetable Barley Soup	70
Progresso Chicken Rice with Vegetables Soup	80
Amy's Alphabet Soup	80
Pacific Chicken Noodle Soup	90
Progresso Vegetable Classics Garden Vegetable Soup	90
Amy's Split Pea Soup	100
Pacific Butternut Squash Bisque	110
Amy's Cream of Tomato Soup	110
Progresso Traditional Manhattan Clam Chowder	110
Pacific Roasted Red Pepper & Tomato Soup	110
Amy's Mushroom Bisque with Porcini	120
Amy's Pasta & 3 Bean Soup	130
Pacific Chicken Spinach Penne Soup	140
Amy's Hearty Minestrone with Vegetables Soup	150
Amy's Summer Corn & Vegetable Soup	150
Progresso Vegetable Classics Lentil Soup	160
Amy's Tuscan Bean & Rice Soup	160
Progresso Hearty New England Clam Chowder	180
Progresso Potato Broccoli & Cheese Chowder	200

* Calories per serving. When the Daily Meal Plan menu specifies soup, have only one serving (8 ounces) unless stated otherwise. (Note cans of soup usually contain about two servings.) See page 223 for additional gluten-free soup manufacturers.

Appendix D
Frozen Food Safety

Increasingly, food giants like ConAgra, Nestlé and others that supply Americans with processed foods concede that they cannot ensure the safety of their food products. Frozen foods can pose a particularly serious safety problem because unsuspecting consumers buy frozen foods for their convenience and incorrectly believe that cooking frozen foods is a matter of taste – not safety.

Still the food industry says that extensive outbreaks of food-borne illness are rare, even though it is well-known that most of the millions of cases of food-borne illness every year go unreported or are not traced to the source. For example, each year approximately 40,000 cases of salmonella poisoning are reported in the United States – but perhaps as many as one million cases go unreported. (Salmonella is a type of bacteria most often found in poultry, eggs, unprocessed milk, meat and water.) Recently salmonella pathogens in some frozen meals have sickened thousands of people.

How could this happen? First, the supply chain for ingredients in processed foods – from flour to fruits and vegetables to flavorings – is becoming more complex and global in the drive to keep food costs down. As a result, government and industry officials concede that almost every food ingredient is now a potential carrier of pathogens. A further complication is that a large number of food companies subcontract processing work to save money and don't require suppliers to test for pathogens. In fact, companies often don't even know who is supplying their ingredients.

In addition, many frozen-food manufacturers have stopped cooking their products at high temperatures, a tactic they call the "kill step," which is intended to eliminate any lingering microbes. Frequently this process step turns some of the frozen food ingredients into mush. So, instead the "kill step" has been shifted to consumers. For example, ConAgra has added food safety instructions to its frozen meals, including the Healthy Choice brand. A typical "frozen-food safety" instruction offers this guidance: "Internal temperature needs to reach 165°F (74°C) as measured by a food thermometer in several spots."

Moreover, General Mills, now advises consumers to avoid microwaves altogether and cook their frozen pizzas only in a conventional oven.

Bottom line: To be safe, always cook frozen foods so that the internal temperature reaches 165°F (74°C) as measured by a good food thermometer.

Appendix E
Exercise Smart

Our bodies are just not built to be immobile and passive. The sad fact, however, is that after years of education and information programs by government agencies, medical associations and insurance companies, relatively few Americans engage in regular
planned exercise – despite the reality that we need to be active to keep our systems working efficiently and rid ourselves of emotional tension. Moreover, exercise burns calories, speeds up your metabolism and is an invaluable part of any weight control program. There are two ways to become more physically active: 1) Increase the physical activity in your daily life; and 2) Start on a regular exercise program. Better still would be a combination of both. Simply stated there are three basic types of exercise: aerobic, stretching and strengthening.

Aerobic Exercises (also called "cardio") condition your cardiovascular system. Aerobic exercises, such as jogging, swimming, cycling, brisk walking, skipping rope, and many others, are typically deep breathing and continuous, with rhythmic and repetitive contractions of your large muscle groups. The trait most aerobic exercises have in common is that they make you work hard and require you process a great deal of oxygen.

Some typical aerobic exercises are: Most strenuous include bicycling, cross-country skiing, dancing (aerobic), hiking in rugged terrain, ice hockey, jogging, jogging in place, rowing, skipping rope, stair climbing, and stationary cycling. Somewhat less strenuous are basketball, field hockey, calisthenics, handball, racquetball, skiing (downhill), soccer, squash, tennis (singles), volleyball, and walking (briskly). Least strenuous aerobic exercises consist of badminton, baseball, bowling, croquet, dancing, gardening, golf (carrying or pulling clubs), horseback riding, housework, ping-pong, shuffleboard, softball, tennis (doubles) and walking (moderate to leisurely).

Stretching-type Exercises such as yoga, tai chi, Pilates and to a lesser extent calisthenics can improve your flexibility – and some of the exercises can make you somewhat stronger.

As you age you inevitably start to loose flexibility. Your gait becomes stiffer; you can't stand quite as upright as you used to; it

becomes tougher to bend over; and you have difficulty turning your neck. Regardless of your age, however, stretching can make you more flexible, less injury prone, and can reduce the pain and discomfort associated with tight muscles and shortened
tendons. Realize, however, that stretching exercises do not condition your heart and lungs. Stretching exercises are fine as long as they are performed in addition to rather than in place of an aerobic exercise.

Most experts do recommend stretching before and after an aerobic or strength routine. However, never stretch cold muscles and always do some form of warm up prior to stretching. Stretch slowly and hold gently. You should stretch to the point of feeling a mild pull, but you should never feel pain. And when you stretch – do not bounce.

Muscle Building and Strengthening Exercises, e.g., weight lifting, use of the machines found in fitness centers and isometrics.

Once more, as you age you loose muscle mass, your bone density decreases and you lose strength. Exercises like weight lifting strengthen your muscles, bones and joints. Strengthening exercises also reduce your risk of developing osteoporosis, a severe bone-loss disease, which can lead to easily fractured bones and all the complications that often follow. Strong muscles not only allow you to lift a sleepy four-year old out of a car without difficulty and lug groceries up to a second floor apartment, but as with increased flexibility, strong muscles also make you less injury prone. Moreover, because **muscle uses many more calories than fat, when you replace fat with muscle, your metabolism actually speeds up.**

For everything you need to know about exercise see *Exercises Smart - U.S. Edition,* an eBook by Earl Simmons also published by NoPaperPress.

NoPaperPress eBooks and Paperbacks

100-Day Super Diet-1200 Cal*
100-Day Super Diet-1500 Cal*
100-Day No-Cooking Diet-1200 Cal*
100-Day No-Cooking Diet-1500 Cal*
90-Day Smart Diet-1200 Cal*
90-Day Smart Diet-1500 Cal*
90-Day No-Cooking Diet - 1200 Cal*
90-Day No-Cooking Diet - 1500 Cal*
90-Day Perfect Diet - 1200 Cal*
90-Day Perfect Diet - 1500 Cal*
60-Day Perfect Diet-1200 Cal*
60-Day Perfect Diet-1500 Cal*
50-Day Flex Diet-1200 Cal*
50-Day Flex Diet-1500 Cal*
30-Day Quick Diet - Women*
30-Day Quick Diet for Men*
30-Day No-Cooking Diet*
30-Day Diet for Women - Metric*
30-Day Diet for Men - Metric*
25 Day Easy Diet-1200 Cal*
25 Day Easy Diet-1500 Cal*
25-Day No-Cooking Diet
10-Day Express Diet
10-Day No-Cooking Diet*
7-Day Diet for Women*
7-Day Diet for Men*
7-Day No-Cooking Diets*
90-Day Gluten-Free Diet-1200 Cal*
90-Day Gluten-Free Diet-1500 Cal*
30-Day Gluten-Free Quick Diet*
30-Day Gluten-Free No-Cooking Diet*
7-Day Diet for Women - Metric*
7-Day Diet for Men - Metric
7-Day Gluten-Free Express Diet*
7-Day Gluten-Free No-Cooking Diet*
90-Day Vegetarian Diet-1200 Cal*
90-Day Vegetarian Diet-1500 Cal*
30-Day Vegetarian Diet*
7-Day Vegetarian Diet*
Weight Loss for Women*
Weight Loss for Women - Metric
Weight Loss for Women - UK
Weight Loss for Men*
Maximum Weight Loss - 1200 Cal*
Maximum Weight Loss - 1500 Cal*

Weight Loss for Men - Metric*
Maximum Weight Loss- 1200 Cal*
Maximum Weight Loss- 1500 Cal*
Weight Control - U.S. Edition*
Weight Control - Metric. Edition
Professional Weight Control Women - U.S.
Professional Weight Control Women - Metric
Professional Weight Control Men - U.S.
Professional Weight Control Men - Metric
Weight Maintenance - U.S. Ed*
Weight Maintenance - Metric. Ed*
Weight Maintenance - UK Ed
Weight Loss for Senior Men*
Weight Loss for Senior Women*
Eat Smart - U.S. Edition*
Eat Smart - Metric Edition
30-Day Mediterranean Diet
Exercise Smart - U.S. Edition*
Exercise Smart - Metric Edition
Exercise Smart - UK Edition*
Total Fitness - U.S. Edition
Total Fitness - Metric Edition
Total Fitness - UK Edition
Total Fitness for Women-U.S. Ed*
Total Fitness for Women - Metric
Total Fitness for Women - UK Ed
Total Fitness for Men - U.S. Ed*
Total Fitness for Men- Metric Ed*
Total Fitness for Men - UK Ed
Senior Fitness - U.S. Edition*
Senior Fitness - Metric Edition*
Senior Fitness - UK Edition*
Computer Diet - U.S. Edition*
Computer Diet - Metric Ed*
Reliable Weight Loss - U.S. Ed
101 Weight Loss Tips*
101 Healthy Eating Tips*
101 Lifelong Fitness Tips*
101 Weight Maintenance Tips
101 Weight Loss Recipes
101 GF Weight Loss Recipes
101 Veggie Weight Loss Recipes*
30-Day Mediterranean Diet*
90-Day Med Diet - 1200 Cal*
90-Day Med Diet - 1500 Cal*

* These titles are available as both ebooks and paperbacks. Our ebooks are sold by Amazon, Apple, Google, Barnes & Noble and Kobo, but our paperbacks are only sold by Amazon.

Disclaimer

This book offers general meal planning, nutrition and weight control information. It is not a medical manual and the authors do not claim to be medically qualified. Everyone should have a medical checkup before beginning this gluten-free weight loss program. Moreover, the physician conducting the medical exam should be made aware of and should approve this diet. Because commercial food ingredients and formulations can change at any time, adults with celiac disease or gluten sensitivity should be particularly careful and double check the ingredients in the foods listed in this book to be sure they are gluten free. We recommend that you do not solely rely on the information presented here and that you always read labels, warnings, and directions before using or consuming a food. For additional information about a product, please contact the manufacturer. The content on this site is for reference purposes and is not intended to substitute for advice given by a physician, pharmacist, or other licensed health-care professional. You should not use this information as self-diagnosis or for treating a health problem or disease. Contact your health-care provider immediately if you suspect that you have a medical problem. Additionally, while the authors and publisher have made every effort to ensure the accuracy of the information in this book, they make no representations or warranties regarding its accuracy or completeness. Further, neither the authors nor publisher assume liability for any medical problems that might result from applying the methods in this book, or for any loss of profit, or any other commercial damages, including but not limited to special, incidental, consequential or other damages, and any such liability is hereby expressly disclaimed.